The National Council Licensure Examination for Practical Nurses

The National Council Licensure Examination for Practical Nurses

Prepared by the National Council of State Boards of Nursing

Eileen McQuaid Dvorak, Ph.D, R.N.

Ray E. Showalter, M.S., R.N.

with review of questions and rationale for the third edition by

Sally A. Black, M.S., R.N.

Jacqueline F. Mitchell, B.S., R.N.

Laura S. Mueller, M.S.N., R.N.C.

Nayereh Shahinpour, M.S.N., R.N.

Susan Szczesny, M.S., R.N.

Joan M. Voluz, M.S., R.N.

Chicago Review Press • 814 N. Franklin St. • Chicago, Illinois 60610

Library of Congress Cataloging in Publication Data
Dvorak, Eileen McQuaid,
  The National Council licensure examination for practical nurses.

  1. Practical nursing—Examinations, questions, etc. 2. National Council of State Boards of Nursing (U.S.)—Examinations—Study guides.
I. Showalter, Ray E., 1929-   . II. National Council of State Boards of Nursing (U.S.)   III. Title.
[DNLM: 1. Licensure, Nursing—United States—examination questions. 2. Nusing, Practical—examination questions. WY 18 D988n]

RT62.D86   1985   610.73'06'93076   85-15003
ISBN 9-914091-66-2

Copyright © 1985 by the National Council of State Boards of Nursing, Inc.

All rights reserved

Printed in the United States of America

Second Edition

The clinical situations described in the test in this book are entirely fictional.
No resemblance to real people or actual medical cases is intended.

Published by Chicago Review Press, 814 N. Franklin St., Chicago, IL 60610

ISBN 0-914091-66-2

Contents

Acknowledgments   1

Introduction   2

General Instructions   22

The National Council Licensure Examination for Practical Nurses

   Part I   23

   Part II   63

Appendix

   Examination Testing Dates   101

   Constructing the National Council Licensure Examinations   102

   State and Territorial Boards of Nursing and Practical Nursing   104

   The Test Plan   109

Acknowledgments

The contributions of many have resulted in the production of the three editions of this book. In the early editions, we acknowledged the support and guidance of the National Council of State Boards of Nursing delegates, Board of Directors and Examination Committee. Recognition of that support and guidance for this new edition continues unabated.

Special recognition to Donald W. Dvorak and to Patricia A. Beck for invaluable assistance in producing the first book for candidates is reiterated here. Their help resulted in the presentation of material in concise and easily understood language.

Producing this new edition has involved assistance from clinical specialists at Rush University Center for Nursing. A special thanks goes to Luther Christman, Dean, College of Nursing at Rush, for recommending members for this group. Thanks also to the staff of the National Council and particularly to David Heidorn, National Council Director of Information Services, for his hours of work in editing, supervising production, and collaborating with the publisher's staff.

One of the authors of the earlier editions was Ray E. Showalter who died in August 1984. Ray's many contributions to the book continue in this edition. One of his last activities at work was chairing the session of clinical specialists in which they reviewed test question content and prepared rationales. His help, as always, was priceless.

A final word of appreciation is given to all those candidates who in the past contributed to the information about the questions presented to assure accuracy and pertinence.

EILEEN MCQUAID DVORAK
Executive Director

Introduction

This book is designed to provide you, a candidate for practical or vocational nurse licensure, with as much information as possible about the examination you must take as part of the process of becoming licensed to practice practical nursing in the United States. (Throughout this book, the term practical nursing will be used to represent practical and vocational nursing.)

The examination is the National Council Licensure Examination for Practical Nurses, more commonly known as NCLEX-PN, and it is administered by member boards of nursing in all but one of the United States, in the District of Columbia, and in the U.S. territories of Guam, the Virgin Islands and American Samoa, all of which will be referred to in this book as states for the purpose of simplicity. At present, California is the only state that does not administer NCLEX-PN.

The organization responsible for preparing NCLEX-PN and its counterpart for registered nurses—the National Council Licensure Examination for Registered Nurses (NCLEX-RN)—is the National Council of State Boards of Nursing, Inc. Founded in 1978, the National Council consists of sixty Member Boards of Nursing, each of whom has been given responsibility by a state legislature to regulate either all nursing practice within a state or, in the case of seven states with two separate boards of nursing, only registered or practical nursing. That responsibility includes not only regulating the practice of nurses already licensed but also regulating the process that determines who may enter into the practice of nursing.

Entry into the practice of nursing, as with any licensed profession, is regulated by states for the purpose of protecting the public from those who are unable to practice nursing safely and effectively. Therefore, candidates for licensure are asked by boards of nursing to provide evidence of their ability to deliver effective nursing care. The primary evidence required is proof of having successfully completed a board-approved

A General Description of the NCLEX-PN

The National Council of State Boards of Nursing and NCLEX

education program and achieving a passing score on NCLEX-PN.

Under the direction of its Member Boards, the National Council developed NCLEX-PN to test a licensure candidate's capabilities to practice safe and effective practical nursing. It is designed to test essential practical nursing knowledge by asking you to apply that knowledge to health care situations demanding practical nursing intervention.

You are already probably well-prepared for such an examination. You have completed a course of instruction in a practical nursing program in which you were taught the basic information necessary to practice safe and effective practical nursing. This was done through various classroom activities, clinical practice, your own study, and examinations constructed to determine whether you had acquired the necessary knowledge and developed an understanding of clinical practice.

That education process is an excellent preparation for NCLEX-PN. The NCLEX examinations are written by faculty members from nursing education programs around the country and clinical practitioners from a full range of practice areas and settings who supervise recently graduated nurses. Some of your own teachers may have been asked, at one time or another, to serve on a writing session for NCLEX-PN.

Basic Information

As to the most basic information about NCLEX-PN, it is a one-day examination given in two time periods of two hours each, one in the morning and one in the afternoon. During each time period, you are provided one of the two test booklets in which the examination questions are printed and responses are written. There are no separate answer sheets. You are allowed to work only in the booklet provided in each time period. The entire examination consists of about 250 questions.

NCLEX-PN is given twice a year, in April and October. Scheduled dates through 1994 are provided in the Appendix. All states administer the examination on the same dates but in test sites selected by each state. Many states use more than one test site, with candidates being assigned to regional locations.

Each state board of nursing establishes its own cut-off dates for applying to take NCLEX-PN and has its own application process with firm deadlines that must be followed by each candidate. You alone are responsible for knowing this information and must request admission to the examination by first contacting the board of nursing of the state in which you seek to be licensed. A list of all the boards of nursing is included in the Appendix.

After the examination is administered, the test booklets are scored by the National Council's test service. While the National Council recommends a specific passing score to its Member Boards, each state exercises its own responsibility for establishing a passing score. The test service reports scores to the state board of nursing or other appropriate agency, and it is the state board or agency that will, in turn, notify you of your score.

Preparing for NCLEX-PN

The NCLEX exam is intended to measure the abilities required for nursing practice. It is not, however, intended to terrify you. It is natural to have the jitters when you are facing an exam that is so important to your future. But you will feel reassured if you remember that what you have learned in nursing school should provide the necessary preparation for taking the NCLEX. You probably know much more than you think you do at this moment.

As a candidate for licensing, you have completed a state-approved program. In the course of your education, you have undoubtedly taken tests and quizzes. Try to remember that the NCLEX exams are prepared in a way not so different from the way individual teachers prepare tests in the classes you took from them. All of the questions on the NCLEX are multiple choice, and you probably already have plenty of experience with this kind of testing. An example of a multiple choice question is:

Insulin is produced in which of the following glands?

○ Pituitary.
○ Pancreas.
○ Ovary.
○ Adrenal.

The first part of this example, which presents the question being asked, is called the *stem*. The stem is followed by four possible answers each preceded by a circle, one of which will be blackened in to show the correct answer. (In this book's sample examination, the circles are labeled ①, ②, ③, ④; on the actual examination, possible answers are not numbered.) One of these four choices provides the correct answer to the question posed in the stem. The other three choices, which are not correct, are called *distractors*. In this example, the correct answer is "Pancreas." The other answers are distractors. To answer the question, you need only to select the number of the correct answer out of the four possible answers given.

You can approach the NCLEX confidently as long as you remember that the exam is not intended to embarrass you or trip you up, but to give you an opportunity to demonstrate the knowledge you have already gained in your study. Most candidates will probably want to do some reviewing for the exam, and this is entirely appropriate.

What to Study?

The best preparation is likely to begin with a review of the textbooks and class notes that you used in your nursing program. Look over old exams and quizzes you have taken in your classes, and review material you found difficult to master when it was first presented. You may discover that material that was difficult when you first studied it is much easier to understand now. After you have identified the gaps in your knowledge, plan to go over that material several times in your review.

Plan from the very beginning of your review to become thoroughly familiar with nursing fundamentals. The questions on the exam will test your ability to apply the basic principles of nursing to a wide variety of clinical situations. Don't let unfamiliar details or terms throw you off the track: always look for the basic nursing principles that are being tested.

How to Review

How to review is to a large extent a personal matter. Think about how you have reviewed for tests in the past. Reading textbooks and notes is one obvious approach. However, tackling those books and notes will be a dismaying task unless you take some time to plan the order in which you will look over the material. Make a brief timetable for yourself, listing topics in the order you want to go over them and allowing more time for difficult topics or topics you studied longer ago. Break your study into manageable parts, rather than simply beginning with your first notebook and plowing right through.

A possibility you may find quite useful is forming a study group with others preparing to take the exam when you do. A study group can be an excellent way to review, but only if everyone is serious about the task at hand and is willing to do the work that will contribute to the group. A study group offers companionship, which is a good way to break the tension everyone feels about the exam. But more than that, if the group members are mature, well-motivated students, each one can lead review sessions in his or her strongest subjects, and the group can tackle the somewhat daunting problem of planning the order in which topics should be reviewed.

Your study group, might, in fact, want to center their review sessions around the practice test in this book. You can examine the questions together and work together to find out why wrong answers are wrong, and why correct answers are correct. As you become more familiar with the kind of questions that appear on the exam, you can formulate similar questions of your own with which to test each other.

Even if you prefer to review on your own, or find it impossible to get together with other candidates because you commute to school or have been out of school for several years, you will still find that this sample test is a valuable study tool. The first time you go over these questions, you should answer them as if you were taking the real examination in the actual time allowed for each section. This will give you a chance to get the "feel" of NCLEX-PN. Be sure to time yourself to see if you are working at the proper pace.

After the initial use of the questions here as a practice examination, the same questions can serve as a basis for review. Consider each question carefully, especially the ones you missed. Decide what the question is asking. If you did not answer it correctly, consider why the answer you chose was not the right one. You may need to return to your textbooks to find material that supports the right answer. For questions you answered correctly, consider what other questions could be asked about that nursing situation and how you would answer these other questions.

Opposite each question, in the right hand column of each page, is a brief "rationale" for the right answer. These brief explanations have been written by clinical practitioners like those who write the questions for NCLEX-PN. Compare your own rationale with those written by these experts. You may be surprised at how much you know. If you know why an answer is correct, consider what other questions could be asked about the nursing situation and how you would answer these further questions. If you do not understand a question or the rationale, that may indicate a gap in your nursing knowledge, and you will want to go back to your textbooks or study group for review of that topic.

These suggestions are just that: suggestions. Trust your own study habits if they have served you well in the past. Remember that the fact you have graduated from an approved educational practical nursing program indicates that you already have a valuable set of study skills.

How Long to Review?

The amount of time needed for review varies. If you have always gotten good grades in your classes and clinical work, and you feel that you understand basic nursing well, then little review may be necessary. Again, your performance on this practice test will give you a good idea about how well prepared you are. If, on the other hand, you know you have serious weaknesses in your knowledge, and you have always felt that you do not know how to study effectively, then you will want to devote several weeks or months to review. The important consideration is to allow yourself enough time to go over the material slowly and carefully, without a feeling of panic. Nothing is harder than mastering material when you feel you have to cram. Plan your review to take as long as necessary and force yourself to stick to your schedule, reviewing a little each day or each week, rather than doing it all in marathon study sessions.

However long your review is, plan to end it a day or two before the exam. You might even go to a movie the night before the test to avoid increasing the tension that often accompanies important exams. Plan to get a good night's sleep, and avoid the temptation to do just a little more cramming. You might learn a few more facts, but you will also make yourself more anxious. Better just to trust your review and your basic knowledge of nursing to see you through.

Are Review Courses Helpful?

Review courses can be helpful. It all depends on you. If you have good study skills and a good grasp of the required material, you should be able to do your own review without taking any courses. Certainly the exam is not conceived with the assumption that candidates will need a review course to pass. However, if you feel the need to have your review structured for you, and you do not trust yourself to keep a study schedule on your own, a review course may be helpful. In selecting a review course, look for one offered by or recommended by your school. Above all, seek one that will provide you with a good overview of basic practical nursing.

How to take NCLEX-PN

Think ahead to the actual day of the exam. Imagine that you have completed your review and feel confident that you are well prepared. You enter the auditorium or classroom where the exam is to be given, and you wait to be seated and given a test booklet.

A skillful test-taker knows that this is not the time to become complacent. Remaining clear-headed and listening carefully to instructions can make a great difference in your performance on the exam. The instructions for taking the NCLEX will be printed in the test booklet, and the proctor will read them aloud, asking you to follow along.

The practice test in this book begins with a copy of the instructions that have been used with past NCLEX exams. Reading these instructions will make you familiar with what you will be expected to do on the exam. However, the instructions for the NCLEX are revised periodically, and the instructions in your test booklet could be slightly different from those here. Don't *assume* that you already know what the instructions will be. Read the instructions carefully before you begin the exam.

Your next concern before actually beginning the exam is to make sure that you understand the time limits. Plan to wear a watch to the exam, even though there probably will be a clock clearly visible in the room. The practical nursing exam is given in two parts, each part taking two hours. The proctor for your exam will probably announce when the time is half gone, or perhaps announce at regular intervals how much time remains.

The exams are planned so that you will be expected to answer between 120 and 125 questions in two hours. This allows you about one minute per question, time enough to read each one carefully and consider your answer, but not enough time to hesitate for several minutes over one question. The best strategy is to go through all the questions first, answering those you are sure of and can answer easily. This will ensure that you will get credit for all the questions you can answer correctly in the time allowed, whether they are at the beginning or end of the exam.

If you use this approach, you may have time left before two hours are up in which to check your answers or to go back and spend extra time on questions you did not know how to answer at first.

After a lunch break (the arrangements will differ according to the state in which you take the exam), you will be allowed another two hours to complete Part II of the exam. Again, you should use the same strategy, going through all the questions first and then going back over the more difficult ones. You may be a bit more tired as you begin Part II and less able to approach the test with a fresh viewpoint, but you will make up for that with the advantage of being more experienced with the format of the exam and the pace at which you must work.

As you go through the exam make sure you read each clinical situation thoroughly. There may be several questions about each case given, and you will lose time if you have to go back and reread the case each time. It will help if you try to visualize the patient described. For example, the correct answer may not be the same for an infant as it would be for an adult.

The cases are intentionally written to be as vivid and realistic as possible. Each patient has a name, and you will be given as many details as needed about his or her background symptoms. Often brief additional information about a case is given between questions to aid you in understanding the case. Try to visualize yourself actually talking to the patient or carrying out the role of the practical nurse in the case. This will help you to understand the questions clearly.

The questions themselves should be read carefully and interpreted straightforwardly. Do not make assumptions about facts that are not given, and do not try to make the questions more difficult than they really are. None of the questions are intended to trick you, and you should not try to read into a question more than is given.

Perhaps, despite thinking hard about a question, you find yourself puzzled. You feel the choices do not include the answer you would have given. In many nursing situations, there are several courses of action that might be appropriate, but on the NCLEX only *one* of the four choices will be correct. Try to imagine yourself doing each of the choices listed, and try to decide which is the best course of action.

The cases given in the NCLEX-PN consist of common **health** problems. However, even if you have never heard of the condition described, you should be able to get many right answers by applying general principles. For example, the principles of asepsis apply to all patients with wounds or incisions: they do not depend on the specific type of wound or how it came about. In most cases, the general principle will lead you to the right answer.

Most of the questions expect you to apply your knowledge to a particular situation rather than just recalling a memorized fact. Therefore, answering the questions may require some thought. If, after some effort, you still do not know the answer, try to decide if you know some things NOT to do. This might allow you to eliminate some answers.

Remember that there is a difference between real-life nursing and test-taking. In nursing practice you obviously cannot act on partial information, guesses, or similarities. But on a test, the fact that your knowledge is not complete should not stop you from using your best judgment. Again, you will feel much more confident approaching the exam if you are familiar with the basics of nursing and trust them to lead you to the correct answer.

Should I Guess on NCLEX-PN?

This is the question all standardized test-takers ask. It will be to your advantage to answer every question because NCLEX-PN is scored by counting correct answers. Unlike some examinations, NCLEX-PN does not have a correction for guessing, which means that no points are subtracted for wrong answers. Even if you answer with a pure guess, you will have a 25% chance of getting the right answer. On the other hand, if you do not answer at all you will have a 0% chance.

However, the psychological aspects of guessing will remain the same. You will *always* increase your chances of getting a right answer if you can eliminate one or two choices as being wrong. Guess, but make educated guesses.

Finally, as you plan for NCLEX-PN, you need to consider what is involved in recording your answers. There is no separate answer sheet for NCLEX-PN. Answers are recorded directly in the test booklet. Do not use the booklet for scratch paper or notes to yourself. The example at the right shows how questions appear in the test booklet.

Use only a number 2 pencil and fill in completely the circle next to the answer you choose, being careful to erase completely any stray marks or responses you wish to change.

Rose, 2 years old, is to receive an antibiotic orally in liquid form. Before pouring the medication, it is essential for the nurse to

○ wipe the lip of the container with a sterile cotton ball.

○ hold the bottle under warm running water for a few seconds.

○ find out if Rose has ever taken a liquid medication.

○ shake the bottle well if there is a precipitate.

Foreign-Educated Nurses

Foreign-educated nurses have much to contribute to health care in this country. After all, the United States has always embraced a diversity of nationalities. Your special outlook and experiences as a foreign-educated nurse can be an advantage as long as your education has provided you with skills equivalent to those of nursing candidates from American programs.

The main purpose of the licensure examination is to protect the public. Passing the licensure examination shows that you are capable of delivering safe and effective nursing care to the public in the United States regardless of where you were educated. The diversity and welcome variation that you as a foreign-educated nurse bring to the public must be considered *after* you have given evidence of your ability to deliver effective nursing care. For you, the licensure exam is particularly important.

You will have several major questions about qualifying to practice at the practical nursing level in the United States. Practical nursing may be a new term for you. In the United States, laws define two forms of nursing practice: registered nurse and licensed practical nurse. You may not have had the same definition of nursing practice where you were educated.

Generally, fine distinctions in judgment are not required of the practical nurse as compared to those required of the registered nurse. And, according to many state laws, the practical nurse functions only under supervision of the registered nurse or other legally authorized professionals.

In many countries the person who performs the same function as the practical nurse in the United States may have a different title. If you have completed a program in another country that you believe prepares you to function as a practical nurse, you will need to present certain documents to the board of nursing in the state where you wish to practice. Most state boards will want evidence of what you studied, how long the program was, how much education you had prior to entering the nursing program, and a copy of the credential or diploma that was awarded when you completed the program. The board of nursing will describe the form of evidence you must give them.

In approximately one-fourth of the states in the United States, a person who completes part of a program for registered nurses may apply for a license as a practical nurse on the basis of equivalent preparation. Also, those candidates for registered nurse licensure who are unsuccessful sometimes find that they can complete requirements for a licensed practical nurse using the basis of equivalent preparation. This, therefore, is an option you might investigate through the state board of nursing where you wish to practice.

You may also wonder if other aspects of nursing are some-

Role of Cultural Differences

what different in the United States. According to studies on the subject, you may find a different emphasis here than in the country where you were educated. Cultural differences may have some impact on your perception of patient needs. The section of this introduction describing the content of the examination and what sample questions are testing should help you to determine if this will be a problem for you. In addition, after trying the sample examination in this book, review each question and correct answer to determine if cultural differences may have had an impact on your choice of answers.

If you find that this is a problem, review with United States-educated nurses or faculty to try to understand the attitudes of people here in the United States for whom you will be expected to give care. Being able to give safe and effective care to people from a cultural background different from yours may be a problem for you, but it cannot be made the problem of the person seeking help—the patient. Again, courses in local schools may be of some assistance.

Besides the possibility of cultural differences, if you do not know English well, you may become worried about the reading difficulty of the licensure examination. Those who develop the examination are aware of the need to keep the reading difficulty as low as possible. There are terms used in nursing that nurses are supposed to know and these are used. Nontechnical words are reviewed with the understanding that the test is not a test of reading ability. Vocabulary is made as easy as possible. The estimated reading difficulty of the examination is the 8th grade reading level.

To understand what this means, compare this practice exam to practical nursing textbooks in English. Most of the current textbooks are at the 10th grade reading level. If you find that you can understand the language used in the textbooks without difficulty, you will probably not find the level of reading in the examination difficult. Of course, the best check on the reading level of the exam is to look at the test questions contained in this book. If the wording of the questions is difficult for you, your proficiency in English may be a problem in taking your licensure examination.

This book describes the examination you will take and gives you a sample test. The questions are all multiple choice. The sections of this introduction on how to study for the test should be reviewed in detail. Review courses also give some assistance. If, after reviewing the sample test in this book, you find you are unfamiliar with this type of testing, you may wish to select a review course offered by a local institution. Courses on how to take a multiple choice test may be particularly helpful if you have not taken this kind of test before.

The other suggestions contained in this book for preparing

for the examinations can be used by you as well as by candidates who completed a nursing program in the United States. The suggestions for study are valuable for all candidates. Generally, additional information on extra assistance by tutors or on review classes can be obtained through the state board of nursing in your state.

The Process of Developing the Examination

Think for a minute about the standardized tests you have taken during your years in school. Where do the questions on these tests come from? Well, you answer, you have never thought about it or you always thought that they just came out of computers or something. It helps to humanize such tests if you realize that the questions were written by real people.

The National Council Licensure Examinations, both NCLEX-PN and NCLEX-RN, are developed with the help of all the state boards of nursing. The National Council has placed responsibility for the development of the examinations in its Examination Committee, which is composed of individuals who are either board members or staff members of Member Boards of Nursing. There are representatives of the four regions of the country—West, South, Midwest and Northeast—on the committee at all times.

Look for the flow chart in the Appendix which shows how the exams are developed. As the first step in the process of developing an examination, as you can see, the members of the Examination Committee prepare what is called a test plan for the examination—one for NCLEX-RN and one for NCLEX-PN.

The test plan is an outline of the nursing content to be covered on an examination. Although the questions on the exam are different each time it is given, the same kind of questions are included for every examination, and the nursing knowledge sampled is the same.

NCLEX neither tests your achievement in your nursing education, nor does it require the experience of nurses who have worked for ten years. As a vocational licensure examination, NCLEX must test a candidate's **vocational** capabilities for the first-time, or entry-level, nursing position. That level of nursing capability is determined through periodic studies of the jobs that entry-level nurses are actually performing throughout the United States.

From the information collected in these studies, the Examination Committee constructs a test plan. The test plan is then submitted to the National Council's Delegate Assembly, which is comprised of representatives from each Member Board of Nursing, for their approval.

Item Writers

Following approval of the test plan, the Member Boards of Nursing are invited on a rotating basis to submit names of individuals to write questions, or items. These people are referred to as item writers and may be faculty members from approved nursing programs or clinical specialists who have contact with students or beginning practitioners.

A committee of the National Council's Board of Directors selects groups of item writers yearly on the basis of their credentials, the region of the country they represent, the type of nursing program they represent, and their expertise in a particular field.

The item writers who are selected work for a week with staff of the test service to develop new questions. Common clinical situations are chosen, each of which may yield a series of questions. The questions are checked by the testing service following each item-writing session to make certain that the questions meet examination specifications, are not ethnically or sexually biased, and are grammatically correct. Both the clinically expert item writers on hand at the session and current nursing textbooks and journals must support the intended correct answer.

Panel of Content Experts

After questions are written, a Panel of Content Experts, one each for NCLEX-RN and NCLEX-PN, reviews the new questions to determine that each is accurate, current, related to the job of the entry-level nurse, and that the answer chosen is, in fact, correct. Members of the panel are chosen in much the same way as the writers, by a committee of the National Council's Board of Directors from nominations submitted yearly by Member Boards on a rotating basis.

Each Member Board may also request to review the proposed questions to make the same determinations on how consistent the questions are with nursing practice in their own state as defined by their state's laws and regulations.

Testing New Questions

These questions are then placed in actual NCLEX examinations and answered by actual candidates. They do not count toward passing or failing the exam, but are included purely to collect information about the questions. Your natural reaction might be to worry about having to answer trial questions, but don't be concerned that the time you spend on a try-out question might be taking away from time you need to spend on a real question. The examination has been planned to allow you more than enough time to answer both the real and the trial questions.

Answer every question carefully because there is a need for practical information from you about the newly developed test questions to make sure that they are clearly written and relevant to practical nursing practice. Obtaining responses on trial questions in this way ensures that the nursing content being tested is current in all states and not confined to selected regions. If there is a trend toward a different emphasis in practical nurse practice in one region of the country, it will be reflected in responses to the try-out questions.

Data gained through the experimental items can identify sources of ambiguity by indicating questions for which a large number of candidates picked the same wrong answer. Even though questions are thoroughly reviewed before they are included as experimental questions, occasionally test takers may interpret a question in a way that was not intended when it was written.

Statistical analyses of the trial questions are reviewed by the Panel of Content Experts. If, with a given question, there is a conflict between its statistical quality and the content the panel wishes to emphasize, content takes precedence. But, of course, statistical information is very important. In the end, the crucial consideration is this question: does this question distinguish between a candidate who knows nursing and one who does not? Questions that do not make this distinction are not used.

This system of checks and balances is used to make sure that only questions testing essential knowledge are used. Every effort is made to ensure that the questions are clear and relevant and that they test important content. There are no trick questions. There are no questions with double meanings. There are no unanswerable questions.

Currency of Licensure Examinations

You may wonder about how up-to-date the licensure examination is. Many times people assume that a period of several years occurs between the selection of test content and the administration of the examinations. On the contrary, the Examination Committee members, with the assistance of the staff of the test service, select the questions to be used in each of the examinations only a short time before the examinations are given. Currency of content is a continuing concern. The short time between selection and administration assures that NCLEX-PN and NCLEX-RN are kept current.

The NCLEX-PN Test Plan

Now that you are familiar with the way individual questions are written for NCLEX-PN, you may be curious about the test plan itself and how it came to be.

As of October 1985, NCLEX-PN has a new test plan. The previous test plan for practical nursing, in effect since 1955, was devised as result of a survey in which experts responded to questions concerning what nursing was or ought to be. Although the test plan underwent some editing and modification to reflect changes in nursing, the basic form remained essentially unchanged until implementation of the new test plan.

In 1983, the National Council published a study that updated nursing's knowledge of the current role of the entry-level practical nurse by identifying the actual job activities performed by the entry-level practical nurse. The study also compared those activities to the activities tested by the previous NCLEX-PN test plan. The study, entitled *Practical Nurse Role Delineation and Validation Study for the National Council Licensure Examination for Practical Nurses*, was performed by the National Council's test service, CTB/McGraw-Hill under the leadership of Helen M. Ference, Ph.D., R.N.

From the study's identification of activities, how frequently they are performed, and how necessary they are for safe and effective nursing, the National Council's Examination Committee constructed a test plan that reflected the relative importance of a nurse's capabilities to perform those activities.

While a copy of the test plan is given in the Appendix, the following section provides examples of questions from each of the eight categories of practical nursing activities that form the basic structure of the test plan. Looking at the test plan is useful because it identifies those activities licensure candidates should know to be successful on the examination and provides the relative importance of those activities on the examination.

Category I — Communicating and Participating in Plans of Care

When Anna is ready for discharge, Ms. Garcia asks the nurse what she should do if Anna begins to develop symptoms of croup again. Which of these questions would it be best to ask Ms. Garcia initially?

① "Has anyone ever showed you how to do postural drainage with Anna?"

② "How far from your home is the nearest emergency room?"

③ "Does rocking Anna or singing to her help to relax her?"

④ "Does your bathroom steam up easily when running the hot water?"

See Part II, question 104, for a complete discussion of this item about planning care.

Category II — Administering Special Therapies: Medications/Oxygen

Before oxygen is administered to Ms. Jacobson, it should be humidified for which of these purposes?

① To decrease the concentration of oxygen during respiration.

② To prevent the oxygen from drying the mucous membranes of the respiratory tract.

③ To reduce the pressure of the oxygen to normal before inhalation.

④ To let the water particles carry the dissolved oxygen to the alveoli.

See Part I, question 52, for a complete discussion of this item about oxygen administration.

Category III — Providing for Therapeutic Needs

In Ms. Turner's early postoperative care, it would be most important to take measures to

① improve her respiratory function.

② increase her nutritional intake.

③ establish a routine pattern for urine elimination.

④ promote expulsion of flatus.

See Part I, question 111, for a complete discussion of this question about therapeutic care, which includes postoperative care.

Category IV — Providing for Basic Health Needs

In view of the prescribed diet high in protein and calories for Mr. Powell, which of these menus would be best for him?

① Bacon, lettuce, and tomato sandwich, fruited gelatin dessert with whipped topping, and cola drink.

② Hot roast beef sandwich with gravy, mashed potatoes, green beans, chocolate pudding, and fruit punch.

③ Beefburger patty, cucumber salad, cooked carrots, apple, and orange juice.

④ Macaroni with tomato sauce, spinach, pear, and milk.

See Part I, question 108, for a complete discussion of this question about nutrition, an important category of basic health needs.

Category V — Collecting and Recording Information

Which of these practices is generally unacceptable in recording on a client's chart?

① Using abbreviations.

② Using incomplete sentences or phrases.

③ Making erasures.

④ Recording subjective symptoms.

See Part II, question 109, for a complete discussion of this question about recording information.

Category VI — Maintaining Safety

Before applying heat to Mrs. Kerr's lower back, it is essential to take which of these actions?

① Place a plastic protective covering on the skin before applying the source of heat.

② Apply a thin layer of petrolatum (Vaseline) on the skin before applying the source of heat.

③ Check the temperature of the source of heat.

④ Wrap the source of heat in a towel.

See Part I, question 83, for a discussion of this safety measure.

Category VII — Promoting Hygiene and Self Care

Mr. Walker is to have physical therapy in preparation for discharge. Which of these measures can the licensed practical nurse carry out on the unit to assist Mr. Walker in his rehabilitation program?

① Giving him warm baths with massage to relax his muscles.

② Instructing him to use a cane to help him to walk.

③ Showing him how to do stretching exercises to loosen his joints.

④ Encouraging him to do self care to meet his own daily needs.

See Part I, question 64, for a complete discussion of self care for this client.

Category VIII — Maintaining a Healthy Environment

Ms. Jones is being prepared for surgery later in the morning. The nurse notices that she is wearing a wedding band and engagement ring. Which of the following actions should be taken?

① Have Ms. Jones remove her rings and put them in the locked medicine cabinet.
② Allow Ms. Jones to wear her rings during surgery.
③ Ask Ms. Jones to place the rings in the bedside cabinet.
④ Have Ms. Jones remove her rings and lock them in the hospital safe.

The correct answer to this question is ④.

Background and Technical Information for the Licensure Examination

The National Council Licensure Examinations (NCLEX) were initiated in 1944. At that time they were called the State Board Test Pool Examinations (SBTPE). The title was changed to National Council Licensure Examinations in 1981. The examinations evolved during the years between 1933 and 1950 when cooperative agreements between two major organizations—the American Nurses' Association and the National League of Nursing Education (later the National League for Nursing)—were made to assist the state boards of nurse examiners.

The state boards were responsible for developing and administering a licensing examination for nursing, and they were under pressure to increase the validity and reliability of examinations, as well as to hasten the scoring time. Because of World War II and the resulting need for nurses, it was necessary to streamline the licensing process and yet maintain a valid examination to protect the public from unsafe health care practitioners. However, even prior to World War II, the need to produce examinations that accurately tested nursing competence had united the state boards of nurse examiners in their efforts to develop a uniform national examination.

Four states participated in the first administration of the State Board Test Pool Examination in January 1944. By the middle of 1944, fifteen states were using the newly developed tests. By 1950 all forty-eight states, the District of Columbia, and Hawaii were participating in the SBTPE. Since that time Alaska (1953), Guam (1969), and the Virgin Islands (1961) have initiated the use of the examination. Although Texas used the SBPTE for registered nurse licensure at an early date, it was not used for practical nurse licensure on a continuous basis until 1968, and California discontinued using the SBPTE for practical nurse licensure in 1974.

The practical nurse examination is a comprehensive exam that includes the usual content areas from practical nurse educational programs. This includes medical-surgical nursing, and professional and vocational relationships. Content from basic sciences, nutrition, and pharmacology is also integrated into the exam.

The National Council of State Boards of Nursing maintains a liaison with the organizations that represent practical nursing: the National Association for Practical Nurse Education and Service and the National Federation of Licensed Practical Nurses. In addition, many licensed practical nurses have been appointed to state boards of nurse examiners and provide input to the licensure examination.

How the Examination Is Scored

The practical nursing exam you will take will contain about 250 questions, and each of the two parts will take two hours, for an examination that lasts a total of four hours. After you complete the examination, your test booklet will be collected and sent to the National Council's test service for scoring. There, your raw score will be computed from the total number of correct answers on your exam. This raw score will then be equated to a *standard score* which indicates how you stand in relationship to the passing score set by your state board. Your standard score will range up to 800. Most people score somewhere between 400 and 600.

Your score will be reported to your state board by the test service, and your board in turn will notify you of your score and whether or not you have passed. Each state sets it own cut-off score for the exam, but the National Council recommends to its Member Boards that the standard score of 350 should be the passing score. A score of 350 or above means you passed; a score below 350 represents failure.

Statistical Background

Although this explanation of passing and failing NCLEX-PN seems straightforward enough, you should be aware that sophisticated statistical methods are required to be sure that your score is calculated fairly and that the tests are accurately measuring what they are intended to measure.

Here again, the National Council depends on its test service. The test service is responsible for considering two important statistical factors that determine whether a test is a good one: its *validity* and its *reliability*.

The validity of a score has to do with its accuracy—in the case of NCLEX, does it really measure whether you can be an effective nurse? The reliability of a score has to do with its consistency—in the case of NCLEX, if you took the examination again would you get about the same score? Or, to put it another way, if the practical nursing examination is valid and reliable, adequately prepared practical nurses will get good scores on it, and, if they take it over and over, they will get good scores each time.

The Criterion-Referenced Scoring System

To help ensure that the NCLEX examinations are valid and reliable, the National Council has turned to a criterion-referenced scoring system. Formerly, the NCLEX examinations were scored with what is called a norm-referenced system, which means that each candidate's score is calculated in comparison to the group of scores of all the candidates taking an examination at the same time.

With a criterion-referenced scoring system, a "criterion" or standard judged to represent an acceptable level of competence is set. That is, a minimum score is set to guarantee that a candidate who demonstrates a certain level of nursing knowledge passes the test. In the remote possibility that an entire group of candidates did very well on the examination, they could all be given passing scores. In practice, however, it should be quickly added that the current pass/fail rate has not changed appreciably with the change to criterion-referenced score setting. In essence, the new criterion-referenced system simply provides a safeguard against admitting incompetent candidates to the nursing profession because the test is scored against a standard that represents competence requirements.

You may be worried, as you read this, about how this minimum level of competence is determined, and how the National Council assures that the lowest passing score is arrived at fairly. This is a complicated issue, involving a combination of the judgment of nursing experts together with statistical techniques.

The Angoff Method

The National Council uses a standard-setting process known as the Angoff method,* a commonly used criterion-referenced standard-setting technique. This method depends on a panel of expert judges who review the test questions on the examination. The National Council uses this method because it is a relatively straightforward procedure that tends to yield a reasonable standard. The procedure involves four steps:

1. The selection and convening of a panel of five to eight judges representing nursing generalists and specialists who are current practitioners supervising entry-level nurses.

2. Definition of a minimally competent applicant model. This is done through review of the job analyses of practical nurses. The judges, working together, agree on all characteristics of a minimally competent beginning nurse.

3. Independent judgment of the performance of a minimally competent candidate on all questions in the examination. This step involves each judge taking a copy of the examination and reviewing it question by question, rating each question on the probability that a minimally competent candidate can answer it correctly.

---

*W. H. Angoff, "Scales, Norms and Equivalent Scores" in *Educational Measurement*, 2d ed., ed. R. L. Thorndike (Washington, D.C.: American Council on Education, 1971)

4. Aggregation of the judgments to produce a passing score for the examination. In this step, all judges' estimates for each question will be averaged. The judges may discuss significant discrepancies among themselves. The averages for all questions are then added together to yield the criterion-referenced standard for the examination.

To illustrate this procedure, you can compare the panel of judges to a group of faculty responsible for a course in nursing. First, they define course objectives. Then, they determine the essential knowledge, skills, and abilities that the students must demonstrate to pass the course. Because of the variability in student performance on paper and pencil tests, faculty average the results of all tests. The faculty also discuss among themselves and reconcile any issues on which they are divided.

You are right if you feel that this process depends heavily on individual subjective judgments and not simply on "impartial" statistical techniques. It *does* depend on the personal judgments of the panel of experts, as does an examination given by an individual instructor in a nursing course. However, this standard-setting process also involves statistical techniques that help to correct and bring into line the judges' individual decisions. Whatever the difficulties involved in criterion-referenced score setting, the National Council believes this method is necessary to make sure that nurses about to enter practice are competent and safe in the delivery of care to patients.

Candidate Diagnostic Profile

For those candidates who fail NCLEX-PN — or any other standardized test, for that matter — the result itself can be painful enough without the added frustration that comes with not knowing as much as possible about why the failure occurred.

To provide information that can help a licensure candidate focus review efforts in preparation for retaking the examination, the National Council's Examination Committee developed the NCLEX Candidate Diagnostic Profile to accompany each failure candidate's score report.

The Diagnostic Profile is an outline based on the NCLEX-PN test plan. Each question on the examination is coded according to the Test Plan. Boxes representing each category will be marked by an "X" when more than 40% of that category's questions on the examination are answered incorrectly.

In a very small percent of cases, no "X" may appear in any box on the Diagnostic Profile. This means that the candidate is apparently weak in most areas of the test plan but not weak enough to trigger an "X" in any particular area.

GENERAL INSTRUCTIONS

This is Part I of the National Council Licensure Examination, which consists of two parts. Each part is in a separate booklet and consists of approximately 120 questions. Included here are some suggestions to help you do your best on this examination. Each question lists four possible answers. You are to select only one answer for each question. Read each question carefully before you decide which one of the suggested answers is correct. Press firmly on your pencil and darken the circle completely next to your answer choice in the examination booklet. You **MUST** use a No. 2 pencil to mark your answers. Erase any stray marks on the page as the examination will be scored by machine and stray marks may be interpreted as incorrect answers. Do not bend or fold any part of the booklet. Use the page identified as "NOTES" for any calculations or notes you might want to make.

The following is a sample question with the correct answer marked properly.

1. Rose, 2 years old, is to receive an antibiotic orally in liquid form. Before pouring the medication, it is essential for the nurse to do which of the following?

    ○ wipe the lid with a sterile cotton ball

    ○ hold the bottle under warm water

    ○ ask if Rose has ever taken liquid medications

    ● shake the bottle well

The fourth choice is the correct answer, and the circle next to it has been marked.

When marking your answer, darken only one circle for each question. Darken the circle completely. Do NOT use X's or check marks. If you decide to change your answer, erase your original answer thoroughly. If you do not, your new answer may be scored incorrectly. Also erase all stray marks on the page. You **MUST** use a No. 2 pencil to mark your answers.

Incorrect Marks   **Correct Mark**

To do your best on this examination, be sure that you understand the following directions before beginning the examination.

- Read each question carefully.
- Select the correct answer from the four possible choices.
- There is only one correct answer to each question.
- Work in a systematic manner; do not spend too much time on any one question.
- If the answer you might prefer is not included, choose one of those listed. Any question that is not answered will be scored as incorrect.

Follow these directions carefully.

DO NOT TURN THE PAGE UNTIL TOLD TO DO SO

I-3

The National Council Licensure Examination for Practical Nurses

PART I

You will be allowed 2 hours
to complete this part of the examination.

Please begin.

Mr. Morris Samm, a 48-year-old married man, has been using nitroglycerin tablets for several months for relief of angina pectoris.

1. The pain of angina pectoris is caused by

   ① inadequate oxygen supply to the myocardium.

   ② pressure on the diaphragm.

   ③ spasms of the intercostal muscles.

   ④ inefficiency of the mitral valve.

Angina pectoris occurs when myocardium oxygen demand exceeds myocardium oxygen supply. It is caused by a temporary inadequacy of the blood supply to meet the needs of the heart muscle. Correct answer ①.

2. The desired effect of nitroglycerin for Mr. Samm is to

   ① constrict his peripheral blood vessels.

   ② improve his coronary blood flow.

   ③ produce slower and stronger heartbeats.

   ④ increase the rate and depth of respirations.

Nitroglycerin improves coronary blood flow by dilating coronary arteries and intercoronary collateral vessels. It relieves the pain of angina within 1 to 2 minutes. Correct answer ②.

Mr. Samm has attacks of severe chest pain that are not relieved by the nitroglycerin. He is admitted to the hospital with a myocardial infarction. Complete bed rest, oxygen by nasal cannula, anticoagulant therapy, a low-sodium diet, and morphine sulfate q. 4h. p.r.n. are prescribed for him.

3. Mr. Samm had morphine one hour before the nurse starts to give him morning care. When the nurse attempts to turn Mr. Samm, he lies absolutely still, refuses to move, and holds his left shoulder with his hand.

The most justifiable interpretation of this behavior is that Mr. Samm

   ① finds this the most comfortable position.

   ② is protecting himself from his surroundings.

   ③ fears that the pain will recur.

   ④ is indicating that he is chilly.

Fear of pain is a normal reaction for Mr. Samm. The pain of myocardial reaction is so severe the client often believes that he is dying. Correct answer ③.

4. Some of the precautions included in Mr. Samm's care while he is receiving oxygen are necessary because oxygen has which of these characteristics:

① It supports combustion.

② It increases body metabolism.

③ It is toxic to the skin when administered in high concentrations.

④ It is lighter than air.

Oxygen supports combustion. Therefore, necessary precautions such as No Smoking signs should be posted in the room and outside the room. Correct answer ①.

5. While Mr. Samm is receiving the oral anticoagulant, it is important to observe him for evidence of

① hives.

② difficulty in breathing.

③ restlessness.

④ hematuria.

Hemorrhage is the principal adverse reaction of anticoagulant therapy. Therefore, the client should be checked for hematuria by a hemostix. Correct answer ④.

6. The nurse assigned to feed Mr. Samm his breakfast assists him to fill out his menu for the next day. Because he is on a low sodium diet the nurse encourages him to select which of the following foods?

① Cereals and dairy products.

② Bakery products and processed meats.

③ Fresh vegetables and fruits.

④ Canned soups and dried fruits.

The nurse should encourage Mr. Samm to eat foods low in sodium. Fresh fruits and vegetables have less sodium than processed foods. Correct answer ③.

7. Which of these questions should be given greatest consideration in selecting a diversion for Mr. Samm?

① Will it be new to him?

② Will it amuse him?

③ Does it promote relaxation?

④ Does it require mental concentration?

Promoting rest and relaxation is a major therapy goal since relaxation decreases oxygen demands. When the nurse suggests any diversion, the need for relaxation should be considered. Correct answer ③.

Mr. Samm suddenly has another myocardial infarction. His condition is critical.

8. Mr. Samm is a Roman Catholic. His wife says to the nurse, "I want my husband to be anointed, but I don't want to frighten him." Which of these responses by the nurse would be most appropriate?

① "Would you like to talk with a priest about this?"

② "This is a decision you must make yourself."

③ "Perhaps your husband isn't nearly as frightened as you are about death."

④ "If I were you, I wouldn't bring the matter up at this time unless your husband mentions it himself."

Recommending a priest to Ms. Samm is the most appropriate response. A priest can address Ms. Samm's worry about frightening her husband. Correct answer ①.

9. Mr. Samm's pulse is thready. A thready pulse is accurately described as

① slow and irregular.

② slow and forceful.

③ rapid and weak.

④ rapid and bounding.

The most accurate description of thready pulse is a rapid and weak pulse. Another description for thready pulse is a fine, scarcely perceptible pulse. Correct answer ③.

10. To save Mr. Samm's energy when he is acutely ill, the nurse should only ask him questions that

① are open-ended.

② he can answer with one word.

③ will encourage him to understand himself.

④ are leading.

One of the major therapy goals is energy conservation and decreased oxygen consumption. In order to conserve energy, Mr. Samm should be encouraged to answer questions with one word. Correct answer ②.

11. Mr. Samm develops Cheyne-Stokes respirations. Cheyne-Stokes respirations are characterized by

① stertorous, deep, labored breathing.

② shallow respirations, gradually increasing in rate.

③ gradually increasing dyspnea and rapid, deep respirations.

④ alternating periods of irregular breathing and apnea.

Cheyne-Stokes respirations are defined as alternating periods of apnea and hyperapnea. Apnea lasting 10 to 60 seconds is followed by gradually increasing and decreasing respirations. Correct answer ④.

12. Mr. Samm dies. In the care of Mr. Samm's body after his death, which of these measures is necessary?

① Padding body prominences.

② Keeping the body in a side-lying position.

③ Positioning the body to prevent drainage from anal and urethral orifices.

④ Handling the body so as to protect it from disfigurement.

The appearance of Mr. Samm's body will be important to his family. Therefore, the body should be arranged to look as natural as possible, as if the deceased person were sleeping. Correct answer ④.

Ms. Dora Miler, 29 years old, is admitted to the hospital with a suspected incomplete abortion. She has abdominal pain and a moderate amount of vaginal bleeding.

---

13. Ms. Miler is to have a sterile vaginal examination. The nurse understands that this procedure requires asepsis. The nurse may hand the physician instruments by three of the following methods. Which one is the **exception?**

① Using sterile gloves.

② Using bare hands after doing a surgical scrub.

③ Using a sterile towel.

④ Using a transfer forceps that is kept in a container of antiseptic solution.

The rule of surgical asepsis states that sterile to sterile equals sterile. Bare hands, no matter how long they are scrubbed, are clean, not sterile. Equipment handled with bare hands would be considered contaminated. Correct answer ②.

Ms. Miler is scheduled to have a dilatation and curettage (D and C) the next day. Her preoperative prescriptions include secobarbital (Seconal) at bedtime.

---

14. In addition to promoting sleep, Seconal is given to Ms. Miler for which of these purposes?

① To reduce the level of anxiety.

② To lessen bronchial secretions.

③ To decrease the muscle tone of the uterus.

④ To minimize the need for postoperative analgesia.

Seconal is a short acting barbiturate which works as a central nervous system depressant. It is administered to Ms. Miller in preparation for surgery to produce mild sedation, thus reducing her level of anxiety. Correct answer ①.

15. When checking Ms. Miler's chart on the morning of surgery, the nurse finds that there is no operative consent. Which of these actions should the nurse take first?

① Obtain an operative consent form and have Ms. Miler sign it.

② Report the absence of an operative consent to the nurse in charge.

③ Notify the operating room staff that the operative consent has not been obtained.

④ Ask Ms. Miler whether she signed an operative consent form on admission to the hospital.

An operative consent is a legal document which protects the client and the hospital. The charge nurse must be told of its absence since she is responsible for management of client care and insuring that consent is obtained before surgery. Correct answer ②.

16. Ms. Miler receives meperidine (Demerol) hydrochloride and atropine sulfate preoperatively. An important purpose of giving atropine at this time is to

① increase the effect of the Demerol.

② help prevent postoperative hemorrhaging by improving the tone of smooth muscle.

③ prevent postoperative dehydration.

④ reduce the possibility of aspiration of respiratory secretions during surgery.

Atropine sulfate reduces salivation and bronchial secretions. It is administered preoperatively to lessen secretions in the upper respiratory tract and thus decrease the possibility of aspiration into the lungs during surgery. Correct answer ④.

Ms. Miler has a D and C under general anesthesia. She is conscious when she is brought back to her unit.

---

17. As soon as Ms. Miler is brought back to her unit after surgery, it would be most important to check her for

① temperature elevation.

② vaginal bleeding.

③ bladder distention.

④ voluntary leg movements.

After dilatation and curettage it is important to monitor the amount of vaginal bleeding. This is done to assess for the possible complication of postoperative hemorrhage. Correct answer ②.

18. Ms. Miler is instructed in perineal care. It would be most important for Ms. Miler to give herself perineal care at which of these times?

① Every 4 hours for the first 24 hours postoperatively.

② During morning and evening care.

③ After using the toilet.

④ When changing sanitary napkins.

Performing perineal care after each elimination insures thorough cleansing of the perineal area, thus decreasing the possibility of introducing organisms from the bladder or rectum into the vaginal opening. Correct answer ③.

19. The nurse transcribes the prescriptions Ms. Miler's physician has written. These include a laboratory slip for a red blood count, stat. Which of the following ranges per cu. mm. of blood is within normal limits?

① 7,000 to 9,000

② 150,000 to 300,000.

③ 2,500,000 to 3,000,000.

④ 4,500,000 to 5,000,000.

4,500,000 to 5,000,000 cu. mm. is in the normal range for red blood cells in a healthy adult female. Correct answer ④.

20. An iron preparation is prescribed for Ms. Miler. To reduce gastric irritation, she should take the iron preparation at which of these times?

① Before breakfast.

② Between meals.

③ Immediately after meals.

④ At bedtime.

Iron preparations may be irritating to the stomach lining and cause nausea. It is best to take iron immediately after meals since food in the stomach prevents the preparation from coming into direct contact with the gastric mucosa and causing irritation. Correct answer ③.

Mr. Samuel Gayle, 42 years old, has chronic leukemia. He is admitted to the hospital with a recurrence of the symptoms of leukemia. Mr. Gayle has been told that his condition is terminal. Mr. Gayle's orders include bed rest, transfusions of whole blood, and an antiemetic p.r.n.

GO ON TO THE NEXT PAGE.

21. For which of these purposes is Mr. Gayle to be given a blood transfusion?

① To cause a remission of the disease and a sense of well-being.
② To depress bone marrow function and blood clotting time.
③ To provide erythrocytes and hemoglobin.
④ To inhibit formation of white blood cells and immune bodies.

A chronic leukemia client suffers from a decrease in the number of erythrocytes in the bloodstream and, therefore, a lowered hemoglobin level. Blood transfusions are the treatment of choice to increase the erythrocyte count and correct the anemia. Correct answer ③.

22. At the time that the blood transfusion is started, Mr. Gayle is given diphenhydramine hydrochloride (Benadryl) intramuscularly. The purpose of this measure is to

① sedate him for the treatment.
② prevent hemolysis of the blood.
③ permit a more rapid infusion of the blood.
④ minimize a possible reaction to the blood.

A client may have an allergic reaction to receiving a blood transfusion. The blood may contain antibodies that trigger this reaction. Oral administration of an antihistamine, such as diphenhydramine hydrochloride, is a method to minimize such an allergic reaction. Correct answer ④.

23. While giving Mr. Gayle special oral care, the nurse notices that his gums bleed easily. The probable cause of this bleeding is

① a breakdown of red blood cells.
② a lowered platelet count.
③ an overproduction of fibrinogen.
④ a destruction of normal white blood cells.

The primary function of platelets is to control bleeding. Clients with low platelet count must be assessed carefully for signs of bleeding. Correct answer ②.

24. In an attempt to reduce the bleeding of Mr. Gayle's gums, the nurse offers him a flavored ice on a stick. The primary reason for this action is that the frozen liquid

① keeps the mucosa moist.
② cools the mouth.
③ promotes clot formation.
④ causes vasoconstriction.

Vasoconstriction can be brought on by application of ice or other cold material. Vasoconstriction will decrease the amount of bleeding. Correct answer ④.

25. Mr. Gayle complains of nausea and eats poorly. Which of these approaches by the nurse would best promote food intake by Mr. Gayle?

① Serving Mr. Gayle his meals at regular mealtimes and saving uneaten food for his between-meal feedings.

② Explaining the importance of good nutrition to Mr. Gayle and encouraging him to eat foods high in protein.

③ Administering the antiemetic to Mr. Gayle a half hour before meals and offering him a diet of small, bland feedings.

④ Giving the antiemetic at the time Mr. Gayle's meals are served and telling him to eat what he can.

An antiemetic given to Mr. Gayle one half hour before a scheduled meal will take effect by the time the meal is served. Relief of nausea will make Mr. Gayle more interested in eating. Small, bland feedings are least likely to provoke indigestion or nausea. Correct answer ③.

26. Mr. Gayle has been depressed since the physician told him that his condition is terminal. An important basic approach to the client who is depressed is

① responding in a mood that is similar to the client's.

② accepting the client's mood.

③ counterbalancing the client's mood.

④ challenging the client's mood.

The nurse's acceptance of Mr. Gayle's mood identifies it as a valid response to his illness and prognosis. This will help with the client's own acceptance of his response as normal. Correct answer ②.

27. Mr. Gayle says to the nurse, "The doctor told me that my blood condition is too severe to be treated successfully. This probably means that I don't have long to live."

Which of these responses would it be best for the nurse to make?

① "Your condition is serious, Mr. Gayle."

② "You should be thinking about making out a will, Mr. Gayle."

③ "It would be better for you to think of something else, Mr. Gayle."

④ "There is always hope, Mr. Gayle."

Mr. Gayle's comments to the nurse are statements of his understanding of his illness. The nurse's response should confirm his realistic statements without giving false hope or trying to distract him. Correct answer ①.

GO ON TO THE NEXT PAGE.

28. Mr. Gayle has a prescription for acetaminophen (Tylenol) p.r.n. For which of these reasons is Tylenol rather than aspirin given to patients who have leukemia?

① Tylenol is more effective than aspirin in controlling the discomfort caused by this disease.

② Tylenol is absorbed in the stomach more rapidly than aspirin.

③ Aspirin preparations interfere with prothrombin formation.

④ Aspirin preparations have a short therapeutic effect.

Mr. Gayle has leukemia and has already had an episode of bleeding from his gums. It is important to maintain his circulatory status and blood clotting mechanisms. Aspirin interferes with prothrombin formation and ingestion of aspirin may lead to another bleeding esplsode. Correct answer ③.

June Banks, 17 years old, is hospitalized to have a biopsy of a small growth on her right leg.

---

29. The physician orders that June's right leg be shaved and then scrubbed with an antiseptic solution prior to surgery. The purpose of this procedure is to

① sterilize the skin.

② improve circulation to the affected area.

③ avoid contamination of the specimen.

④ reduce the possibility of infection.

The overall goal of the surgical prep is to reduce the chance of infection. Response ① is incorrect because a shave and a prep will only clean the skin, not sterilize it. Correct answer ④.

30. While the nurse is preparing June's leg for the biopsy, June says, "If this lump turns out to be cancer, what happens next?" Which of these responses by the nurse would be most appropriate?

① "I can't say. It's really hard to know exactly what will happen."

② "I know you're worried. Have you spoken with your doctor about it?"

③ "What makes you think that you might have cancer?"

④ "It's best to wait until after the biopsy to find out if it's cancer."

The nurse should acknowledge June's anxiety and allow June to explore the options her physician has already identified. Correct answer ②.

The biopsy is performed and the results indicate that a malignancy is present. The physician informs June and her parents of the results of the biopsy. June is scheduled for a below-the-knee amputation of her right leg.

31. At 2 a.m. on the morning of surgery, the nurse finds June awake and crying. In addition to notifying the nurse in charge, which of these actions should the nurse take?

① Review with June the procedures that are to occur later that day.

② Give June a back rub.

③ Remind June that she needs her sleep in preparation for the operation.

④ Encourage June to read a favorite magazine until she gets drowsy.

Early on the morning of surgery, it is most important for June to be relaxed. By now June has probably done enough talking about the procedure. A back rub will provide a way for the nurse to offer nonverbal comfort and relax June so she can sleep. Correct answer ②.

32. June is being transferred to a stretcher to go to the operating room. Which of these illustrations shows the best position for the nurse when assisting June in moving from the bed to the stretcher?

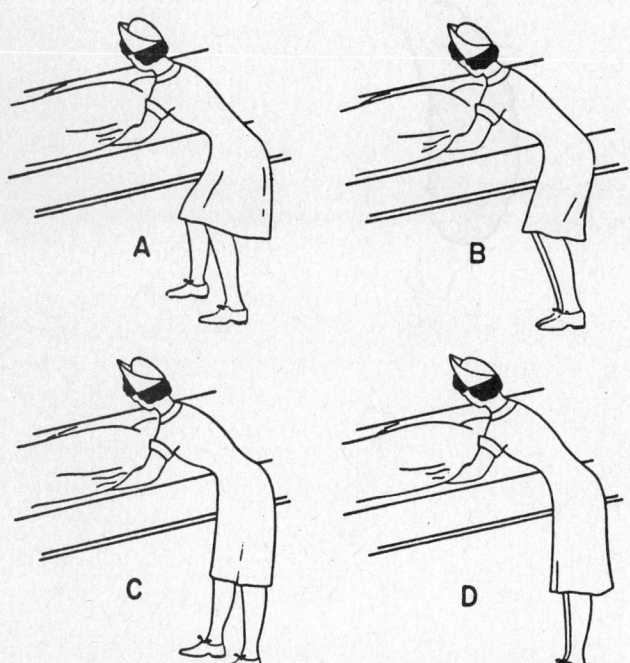

① A.
② B.
③ C.
④ D.

Picture A illustrates the best body mechanics. Bending the knees and keeping the feet apart protect the nurse's back. Correct answer ①.

33   GO ON TO THE NEXT PAGE.

June has a below-the-knee amputation of her right leg as planned. After the surgery, she is brought to the recovery room.

33. In addition to monitoring June's vital signs, it is essential to take which of these actions?

① Place her on her left side with pillows supporting the stump.

② Place her on her back with sandbags on either side of the stump.

③ Check her dressing for odor.

④ Check her dressing for bleeding.

In the immediate postoperative period, bleeding is the principal concern. Although position and control of infection are important, they are not a priority at this time. Correct answer ④.

June is transferred to the adolescent unit.

34. On June's second postoperative day, physical therapy is prescribed for her. Two days later, she refuses her breakfast and lies in bed with her face turned toward the wall. When the nurse who is assigned to take June to physical therapy goes into her room, June refuses to move or to acknowledge the nurse's presence.

Which of these comments would it be best for the nurse to make first?

① "It's important for you to go for treatment now, June."

② "You have to stop feeling sorry for yourself if you want to get better, June."

③ "Would you rather have someone else help you, June?"

④ "Can you tell me what's bothering you, June?"

A grief reaction should be expected following an amputation. "Can you tell me what's bothering you, June?" acknowledges June's grief and is not judgmental or punitive. Correct answer ④.

35. In the postoperative period, June's diet should be high in

① vitamin C and protein.

② vitamin D and carbohydrate.

③ iron and magnesium.

④ calcium and phosphorus.

Vitamin C and protein are needed to promote adequate wound healing and should therefore be plentiful in June's diet. Correct answer ①.

36. The nurse understands that adjusting to amputation is difficult for any client, and especially so for June because 17-year-olds characteristically

① have frequent mood swings.
② have difficulty expressing their feelings verbally.
③ need to be like their peers.
④ need to be physically active.

Adolescents need the social approval of their peer group, and June's concern about her friends' acceptance will cause added difficulty in her adjustment to the amputation. Correct answer ③.

37. June demands a great deal of attention from the nursing staff and frequently puts her call light on to complain bitterly about her care. When the nurse enters her room one evening to prepare her for the night, June says, "What the hell's going on out there? Why can't I get somebody in here?"

Which of these responses should the nurse make first?

① "Everyone has to wait her turn, June. Now that I'm here, what would you like me to do?"
② "You sound terribly unhappy, June. I'll be glad to do what I can to help you."
③ "We're doing our best, June, but there are many patients here who are really ill."
④ "You must be more understanding, June. We answer your call light as quickly as we can."

The nurse should be sensitive to the underlying reason for June's outburst. June is scared, unhappy and depressed. All the other answers are wrong because they do not acknowledge June's feelings and instead require June to understand the pressures of the nurse's job. Correct answer ②.

38. Which of these actions should be taken if June experiences phantom-limb sensation?

① Exercise the stump.
② Elevate the stump.
③ Divert June's attention.
④ Encourage June to talk about the feeling.

Phantom-limb pain is both physiological and psychological in origin. Pain medication and ventilation of feelings are the accepted treatment. Exercise and elevation will not help. Diverting June's attention may decrease pain perception somewhat, but it is not a definitive treatment. Correct answer ④.

Mr. George Cone and Ms. Mae Foster are elderly and widowed, and are living in a residence that provides supportive services. They have several times been found in each other's rooms, engaged in necking, petting, and sexual intercourse. There is considerable gossip among residents about their behavior.

39. The sexual behavior of Mr. Cone and Ms. Foster is being discussed in a staff meeting. To arrive at a plan of action, it will be most important to have which of these understandings about this couple?

① They are satisfying a physical instinct.

② They are acting rebelliously.

③ They are meeting an emotional need.

④ They are being exhibitionistic.

It is common for elderly clients who have lost a spouse to miss the physical contact and emotional support the spouse formerly provided. Mr. Cone and Ms. Foster are responding to one another's genuine sexual and emotional needs. It is important for the nursing staff to respect these needs before arriving at a plan of action. Correct answer ③.

40. Mr. Cone tells the nurse that he has two full-grown sons. He frequently discusses with the nurse the pros and cons of the way he brought them up, and he often wonders whether they are reasonably happy now.

What is the meaning of Mr. Cone's behavior?

① He is living in the past.

② He is attempting to be entertaining.

③ He is dealing with an unresolved conflict.

④ He is indulging in self-pity.

Mr. Cone's repeated discussions of his child rearing methods illustrate his uncertainty about them. He continues to be uncertain whether he always made appropriate decisions, and wonders whether his children suffered from them. Correct answer ③.

41. In the situation described in the previous question (#40), which of these responses would be best?

① Indicate interest in what Mr. Cone is saying.

② Offer to play a card game with Mr. Cone.

③ Explain to Mr. Cone that it is too late to do anything about that now.

④ Tell Mr. Cone that most fathers worry about such things.

In caring for a client who is dealing with an unresolved conflict, the nurse should recognize the importance of the conflict in the client's mind. Expressing interest in what the client says is one way to offer this recognition. Correct answer ①.

Mr. Cone has severe chest pain and is transferred to the coronary care unit in a nearby hospital. The unit has restricted visiting hours. His prescriptions include an electrocardiogram (EKG).

42. Which of these factors are generally considered to be related to the development of coronary artery disease?

① Drinking moderate amounts of alcoholic beverages and participating in sports that involve vigorous arm movements.

② Being overweight and living under persistent pressure.

③ Having irregular meal hours and living in a climate with marked seasonal variations.

④ Eating a diet high in polyunsaturated fats and getting insufficient sleep.

Coronary artery disease is considered to be related to a person's daily life and habits. Weight also is thought to have an effect on the development of coronary artery disease. An overweight person subjected to stress can be a candidate for developing coronary artery disease. Correct answer ②.

43. Mr. Cone's care should be based on which of these understandings about a client's expected response to being admitted to a critical care unit?

① The complexity of the equipment in the environment will be reassuring and will serve to lessen the client's anxiety.

② The sudden change in environment and the possibility of life-threatening illness will tax the client's usual coping mechanisms.

③ The experience will be nontraumatic if the client has been successful in coping with stresses in the past.

④ The competence of the staff will determine the extent of the psychological effect of the client's stresses.

Mr. Cone's admission to a critical care unit exposes him to new machinery, noises, staff, and medical tests. This new environment and the fear of losing his life will be stressful for him. Mr. Cone may find his usual methods of coping are not adequate for this new level of stress. Correct answer ②.

44. In preparing Mr. Cone for the EKG, the nurse should include which of the following information about the procedure?

① He will have nothing by mouth for 12 hours before the procedure.

② He will have no discomfort during the procedure.

③ He will be required to do mild exercise during the procedure.

④ He will have to remain flat in bed for several hours after the procedure.

Since Mr. Cone is in a totally new environment, his anxiety can be eased by having accurate information provided by the nurse. An EKG has no preparation, no physical exercise requirements and no adverse side effects. Correct answer ②.

GO ON TO THE NEXT PAGE.

A nurse is with Ms. Foster at the residence.

45. Ms. Foster asks the nurse if she can visit Mr. Cone. Which of these responses would be best?

① "I'll have to find out if Mr. Cone wants to see you."
② "I'll call Mr. Cone's unit to see if we can arrange a time."
③ "Mr. Cone will probably be back in a couple of days."
④ "Mr. Cone needs rest more than anything else."

Because Mr. Cone and Ms. Foster are involved in a relationship, it is natural for Ms. Foster to be concerned about Mr. Cone. If the coronary care unit allows visitors, arranging for Ms. Foster to visit will reassure her that Mr. Cone is stable. Correct answer ②.

Mr. Cone's physical condition improves and he is returned to the residence. His prescriptions include a digitalis preparation.

46. Which of these symptoms is an indication of digitalis toxicity?

① Thirst.
② Diuresis.
③ Nausea.
④ Hematuria.

Symptoms of digitalis toxicity include: decrease in pulse, cardiac arrhythmias, nausea, vomiting, loss of appetite, abdominal cramps, visual disturbance and complete heart block. Of the choices here, nausea is the only one recognized as a symptom of digitalis toxicity. Correct answer ③.

Ms. Emma Jacobson, 43 years old, is admitted to the surgical unit. She is scheduled to have a bronchoscopy. Cancer of the lung is suspected.

47. Following the bronchoscopy, it is essential that Ms. Jacobson receive which of these instructions?

① "Call the nurse before you take a drink of anything."
② "Take deep breaths and cough every hour."
③ "Tell us whenever you wish to get out of bed."
④ "Avoid talking for three hours."

After bronchoscopy the nurse must determine the return of the "gag" reflex before the client is allowed to take fluid. If the gag reflex is not present, Ms. Jacobson could aspirate when she takes a drink. Correct answer ①.

48. Which of these symptoms experienced by a client who has just had a bronchoscopy would be most indicative of a serious complication of the procedure?

① Coughing.

② Difficulty in breathing.

③ Hoarseness.

④ Pain when swallowing.

A serious complication of bronchoscopy would be swelling due to the trauma of the procedure. The first symptom the client would experience would be difficulty in breathing. Correct answer ②.

The results of Ms. Jacobson's diagnostic tests indicate that she has cancer of the lung. A lobectomy of her right lung is scheduled and she is informed of her prognosis.

---

49. Ms. Jacobson expresses discouragement about her diagnosis and her surgery. Which of these measures by the nurse would probably provide the most emotional support for Ms. Jacobson?

① Talking to her.

② Encouraging her family to visit.

③ Trying to change her mood.

④ Listening to her attentively.

Before any action can be taken, the nurse must determine what Ms. Jacobson is feeling. Listening attentively will provide emotional support, as well as allowing the nurse to discover whether Ms. Jacobson needs additional help or information. Correct answer ④.

50. Ms. Jacobson will have a chest tube attached to underwater drainage following her surgery. The primary purpose of the chest tube is to

① allow for the removal of fluid and air.

② make deep breathing and coughing easier.

③ prevent rapid re-expansion of the lung.

④ control pulmonary hemorrhage.

A chest tube is inserted into the pleural space to allow for the drainage of fluid and air and to maintain a negative pressure. Correct answer ①.

Ms. Jacobson has a lobectomy of her right lung. Following a stay in the recovery room, she is brought back to her unit with a chest tube in place. Ms. Jacobson's orders include morphine sulfate q. 4h. p.r.n., oxygen by nasal cannula, and diet as tolerated.

51. The nurse records in notes about Ms. Jacobson that fluid is fluctuating in the chest tube with each respiration.

Which interpretation of this recorded information is correct?

① Oxygen is being lost through Ms. Jacobson's chest tube.

② There is an air leak within the drainage system.

③ The apparatus is functioning properly.

④ Air is being drawn into Ms. Jacobson's chest cavity.

Fluctuation is expected to occur with each respiration. If fluctuation does not occur it indicates that a blood clot is plugging the tubing or that the lung has reinflated. Correct answer ③.

52. Before oxygen is administered to Ms. Jacobson, it should be humidified for which of these purposes?

① To decrease the concentration of oxygen during respiration.

② To prevent the oxygen from drying the mucous membranes of the respiratory tract.

③ To reduce the pressure of the oxygen to normal before inhalation.

④ To let the water particles carry the dissolved oxygen to the alveoli.

The air we normally breathe carries a certain amount of humidity. When the client is being given a higher concentration of oxygen, it is important to increase the humidity so that the mucous membrane of the respiratory tract does not dry out. Correct answer ②.

53. While Ms. Jacobson is receiving oxygen, three of the following measures may be carried out for her. Which one is **contraindicated**

① Taking her temperature orally.

② Giving her sponge baths.

③ Urging her to drink fluids.

④ Assisting her to deep-breathe and cough.

Oral temperature-taking is contraindicated when Ms. Jacobson is receiving oxygen. The flow of oxygen and the additional humidity will affect the reading. Correct answer ①.

54. All of the following beverages are available for evening nourishment on Ms. Jacobson's unit. Assuming that servings are average, which of these drinks would provide the greatest amount of a vitamin that promotes healing?

① Tea with lemon.

② Apple juice.

③ Tomato juice.

④ Prune juice.

Tomato juice contains high amounts of vitamin C. Vitamin C promotes healing. Correct answer ③.

55. During the evening of the second postoperative day, Ms. Jacobson complains of pain. Which of these actions should the nurse take first?

① Check her chart to ascertain the time of her last dose of medication for pain.

② Report her symptom to the medication nurse.

③ Give her a soothing back rub and change her linen.

④ Ask her to describe her pain.

A complaint of pain can have many causes. First the nurse must determine the specifics by asking Ms. Jacobson to describe her pain in more detail. Correct answer ④.

On Ms. Jacobson's third postoperative day, her temperature begins to rise above the normal level. The physician's prescriptions include a tepid water sponge bath for Ms. Jacobson if her temperature should rise above 102° F. (38.9° C.). At 8 p.m., the nurse takes Ms. Jacobson's temperature. It is 103° F. (39.4° C.).

---

56. In which of these ways is body heat lost through the use of a tepid water sponge bath?

① Production of more perspiration.

② Stimulation of the cold receptor endings in the skin.

③ Penetration of water into the pores to cool the underlying tissues.

④ Evaporation of water from the skin.

A tepid sponge bath will increase the body heat lost through evaporation. A tepid sponge bath will neither increase the perspiration nor penetrate into the pores. Although cold receptors are stimulated, this will not lower body temperature. Correct answer ④.

GO ON TO THE NEXT PAGE.

57. On which of these areas of Ms. Jacobson's body should the nurse place cool, moist cloths during the tepid water sponge bath?

① Groins and axillae.

② Back and neck.

③ Upper and lower extremities.

④ Feet and head.

Arterial blood supply is very superficial at the groin and axillae. Therefore these are effective points on which to place cool cloths. Correct answer ①.

58. Ms. Jacobson is to have increased fluids, but she is reluctant to drink. Which of these measures will probably help most to increase her fluid intake?

① Explaining to her that she will need fluid until her infection has cleared up.

② Offering her a small glass of fluid every hour.

③ Serving her sweetened liquids between meals.

④ Keeping a pitcher of water on her bedside table.

Offering Ms. Jacobson fluids every hour will provide her with a graphic reminder of the importance of adequate fluid intake. In addition, small amounts will not overwhelm Ms. Jacobson, and she is more likely to be able to take the prescribed amount of fluid. Correct answer ②.

Mr. Charles Walker, 57 years old, is being treated for Parkinson's disease. He is admitted to the hospital for a re-evaluation of his condition. His admission prescriptions include diet as tolerated and activity as desired.

---

59. Upon Mr. Walker's admission, which of these measures should be given priority?

① Explaining to him the roles of various nursing personnel.

② Introducing him to long-term ambulatory clients.

③ Finding out about his routines for care at home.

④ Evaluating how much he knows about his condition.

Collecting and recording information is an important category of practical nursing activity. Interviewing the client is one method of collecting data. The client is usually the best source for information about his patterns of coping with activities of daily living. Correct answer ③.

60. Which of these statements about clients who have Parkinson's disease is accurate?

① They have transitory memory lapses.

② They have no intellectual impairment.

③ Their emotional liability is temporary.

④ Their mental depression cannot be overcome.

Clients with Parkinson's disease may exhibit impaired judgment, but their IQs are usually within normal limits. These clients may need intellectual stimulation, but that does not imply impairment. Correct answer ②.

61. In planning Mr. Walker's care, **greatest** consideration should be given to

① completing his care in as short a period as possible.

② organizing his care so that he will feel unhurried.

③ encouraging him to assume full responsibility for his care.

④ providing long rest periods for him after each of his care activities.

The first symptoms of Parkinson's disease are usually tremors which tend to become aggravated by stress and anxiety. The client's care should include ways to reduce anxiety-producing situations. By allowing enough time to perform activities, the client will not be rushed, and stress will be lessened. Correct answer ②.

62. Mr. Walker has been receiving levodopa (Larodopa). The purpose of this medication for him is to

① relieve the symptoms of his disease.

② prevent the progression of his disease.

③ promote his resistance to infection associated with his disease.

④ provide him with nutrients lost in abnormal amounts as a result of his disease.

Drug therapy is used for symptomatic treatment, as there is no cure for this disease. Levodopa has been used successfully in reducing tremors and rigidity. Correct answer ①.

63. Mr. Walker is to have an oil retention enema and a cleansing enema. The desired effect of these measures is best achieved if

① the cleansing enema is given before the oil is instilled.

② the cleansing enema is given immediately after the oil is instilled.

③ the oil is given first and remains in the bowel for a period of time before the cleansing enema is given.

④ the oil and the solution for the cleansing enema are mixed thoroughly and given together.

Constipation is sometimes a problem for clients with Parkinson's disease. The order and timing of enemas should be governed by the desired effect. The oil retention enema lubricates the rectum and softens the stool. The cleansing enema stimulates peristalsis through irritation of the colon and rectum. Correct answer ③.

64. Mr. Walker is to have physical therapy in preparation for discharge. Which of these measures can the nurse carry out on the unit to assist Mr. Walker in his rehabilitation program?

① Giving him warm baths with massage to relax his muscles.

② Instructing him to use a cane to help him to walk.

③ Showing him how to do stretching exercises to loosen his joints.

④ Encouraging him to do self-care to meet his own daily needs.

One of the goals in caring for the client with Parkinson's disease is to prolong independence. Therefore, Mr. Walker is encouraged to carry out his usual activities of daily living. Correct answer ④.

65. Mr. Walker is a journalist. One day, after trying to work on a manuscript, Mr. Walker suddenly sweeps the sheets of paper off the overbed table onto the floor. He exclaims disgustedly, "Oh, what's the use?" and starts to cry.

To deal effectively with this situation, the nurse should have which of these understandings about Mr. Walker's behavior?

① A complete knowledge of the effects of an illness by a client insures acceptance of the illness.

② Lack of acceptance of an illness is evidenced by immature actions.

③ Clients with a chronic illness tend to seek sympathy for their condition.

④ Frustration occurs when clients can no longer be independent.

It is natural for Mr. Walker to be frustrated by his inability to work. The nurse might suggest that he rest briefly and then return to his manuscript, thus expressing confidence that he is still capable of independence and productive work. Correct answer ④.

Ms. Laura Riley, 20 years old, goes to a neighborhood clinic because she has a purulent vaginal discharge. The physician suspects that Ms. Riley has gonorrhea. She is to have a pelvic examination.

---

66. The nurse instructs Ms. Riley to empty her bladder prior to the pelvic examination. The **chief** purpose of this instruction is to

① prevent possible rupturing of a distended bladder.

② visualize the vaginal canal more easily.

③ aid in assessment of the pelvic organs.

④ enable the pelvic organs to reassume their normal position.

The bladder lies in the anterior of the pelvis and could, if full, interfere with assessment of other pelvic organs. An emptied bladder also allows for a more relaxed client. Correct answer ③.

The results of the diagnostic tests confirm that Ms. Riley has gonorrhea.

---

67. Which of these medications is generally used in the treatment of gonorrhea?

① Penicillin.

② Streptomycin.

③ Sulfisoxazole (Gantrisin).

④ Neomycin sulfate.

Gonorrhea is a bacterial infection. The medication of choice is penicillin, unless the client is allergic. Penicillin is a relatively low-priced antibiotic with minimum toxicity. Correct answer ①.

68. Because Ms. Riley has gonorrhea, the information is to be reported to the Health Department. The chief purpose of reporting gonorrheal infections to an official health agency is to

① provide for the study of current sexual habits.

② isolate infected individuals during the treatment period.

③ identify possible infected persons.

④ compile statistics on venereal disease.

Because gonorrhea is an infectious venereal disease, Health Departments require that cases be reported in order to control the spread of the disease. When infected persons are identified, their sexual contacts may also receive proper treatment. Correct answer ③.

69. Sterility in women that results from untreated gonorrhea is caused by

① scarring of the cervix.

② cyst formation in the ovaries.

③ strictures of the fallopian tubes.

④ interference with the production of follicle-stimulating hormone (FSH).

If gonorrhea goes untreated, the infection may travel to the fallopian tubes. Here, acute inflammatory changes cause narrowing of the fallopian tubes. Possible complications of these strictures include ectopic pregnancies or sterility. Correct answer ③.

Ms. Riley returns to the clinic for a follow-up visit. She is to have a Papanicolaou (Pap) test.

---

70. The nurse should explain to Ms. Riley that a Pap test is

① a biopsy of the vaginal wall to detect pathologic changes.

② a study of cervical cells to detect atypical cells.

③ a uterine smear to detect endometritis.

④ an examination to detect pelvic infection.

A Pap test specimen is obtained by swabbing secretions from the cervix of the uterus. A microscopic study of the cells that a woman's body normally sheds is used to detect the presence of any abnormal cells. Correct answer ②.

Mr. Victor Little, 82 years old, is admitted to the hospital with benign hypertrophy of the prostate gland. He is scheduled for a transurethral prostatectomy.

---

71. The nurse assigned to admit Mr. Little is able to assess and record his symptoms because the nurse understands that the prostate gland is located

① within the lumen of the urethra.

② within the seminal vesicles.

③ around the testes.

④ around the neck of the bladder.

The prostate gland surrounds the urethra just below the bladder. Correct answer ④.

72. When assessing Mr. Little's symptoms, the nurse asks if he has had difficulty voiding. This symptom of benign prostatic hypertrophy is caused by

① pressure of the prostate gland on other structures.

② infiltration of the prostate gland into other tissue.

③ inflammation of the prostate gland.

④ excessive secretion from the prostate gland.

As the prostate gland enlarges it puts pressure on the urethra causing urinary stasis, recurring infections, frequent urination, nocturia and dysuria. Correct answer ①.

73. Mr. Little's blood is typed and cross matched before surgery. A purpose of typing Mr. Little's blood is to

① determine the ratio of the formed elements in his blood to the plasma.

② estimate the amount of blood he will need.

③ assess his bleeding pattern.

④ identify his Rh factor.

Blood typing determines both blood type and Rh factor for Mr. Little, important information if blood transfusions are to be given during surgery. Correct answer ④.

74. Mr. Little says to the nurse the evening before surgery, "My daughter called my minister, and he was supposed to come to see me this evening. I doubt if he will be coming now—it's eight o'clock already."

Which of these responses would be most appropriate initially?

① "Would you like me to check to see if your minister is still planning to come this evening, Mr. Little?"

② "Your minister keeps his word, Mr. Little. I think he'll come."

③ "Your minister may be planning to come in the morning if he can't visit you this evening."

④ "Since you feel that your minister may not come, would you like to see another minister?"

An appropriate response would be for the nurse to check to see whether Mr. Little's minister is coming. If not, another visit can be arranged. Answers ② and ③ are empty promises and a way of putting Mr. Little off. Correct answer ①.

Mr. Little has a transurethral prostatectomy. When he is returned to the unit, he has an indwelling urethral catheter that is attached to a bedside drainage container. He is to have intermittent bladder irrigations with normal saline solution. An analgesic has been prescribed for him.

75. Which of these understandings should the nurse have about the catheter irrigations for Mr. Little?

① The solution should be at room temperature and allowed to flow in by gravity.

② No more than 50 ml. of saline should be instilled, and a moderate amount of suction should be used to withdraw the solution.

③ The equipment and solution must be sterile, and the solution must be allowed to return by gravity.

④ The procedure should be continued until the returns are clear.

Because the bladder is a sterile area, the solution must be sterile. In addition, the solution should be returned by gravity since increased suction may irritate the operative area and increase bleeding. It would be unrealistic to expect the fluid to be clear so soon after surgery. Correct answer ③.

76. If Mr. Little complains of pain in the bladder area, which of these measures would probably be best first?

① Finding out when he received his last medication for pain.

② Taking his blood pressure.

③ Checking his urinary drainage apparatus.

④ Reporting his complaint to the nurse in charge.

A clogged urinary catheter would be an obvious cause of increased pain after a transurethral prostatectomy. Such a clog could be due to the presence of a blood clot. The correct response is to check Mr. Little's urinary drainage apparatus. Correct answer ③.

77. Three of the following measures would be appropriate in taking care of Mr. Little's indwelling urethral catheter. Which one is the **exception**?.

① Having the end of the drainage tubing above the level of the urine in the drainage collection container.

② Arranging the drainage tubing so that accumulation of urine in the bladder will not occur.

③ Keeping the drainage collection container below the level of the bladder.

④ Tucking the connector on the drainage tubing under the edge of the drawsheet while the catheter is being irrigated.

Since the bladder drainage is a closed sterile system, every time the system is opened the sterility must be maintained. Tucking the connector under the drawsheet would contaminate the connector, making it an inappropriate action. Remember, the question asks for the INAPPROPRIATE action. Correct answer ④.

78. The nurse notes that the drainage in Mr. Little's urethral catheter has become bright red and notifies the registered nurse, knowing that the nursing action to be taken will be to

① clamp the urethral catheter.

② elevate the foot of the bed.

③ administer his prescribed analgesic.

④ irrigate his bladder.

Irrigation of the bladder should prevent clot formation and maintain patency of the catheter. Correct answer ④.

79. Which of these measures will be most important during Mr. Little's morning and evening care?

① Encouraging him to do his own care.

② Giving thorough care to his perineal area.

③ Providing him with the equipment necessary for him to administer his perineal care.

④ Instructing him to maintain a high-Fowler's position during bathing.

Mr. Little will require catheter care and strict attention to his perineal area. The nurse must assess the drainage as well. It would be inappropriate for Mr. Little to do this complex care himself. Correct answer ②.

Mr. Little's bladder irrigations are discontinued and he is to start progressive ambulation.

80. Mr. Little is to get out of bed for the first time and is to ambulate. Which of these actions should the nurse take **first**?

① Clamp Mr. Little's urethral catheter.

② Place an armchair along the side of Mr. Little's bed.

③ Have Mr. Little sit on the edge of the bed with his feet on a flat surface.

④ Provide a walker for Mr. Little's use.

After a period of bed rest, Mr. Little will need time to adjust to an upright position. Sitting on the edge of the bed will aid in this adjustment. It would be inappropriate to clamp the urethral catheter at this time. Correct answer ③.

81. After Mr. Little's catheter is removed, which of these conditions is most likely to occur?

① Dribbling of urine.

② Voiding of large amounts of urine.

③ Increased concentration of the urine.

④ Appearance of blood in the urine.

The presence of a urinary catheter dilates the urinary sphincters. After the catheter is removed, it would not be unusual for dribbling of urine to occur. Blood in the urine is possible, but not as likely as dribbling. Correct answer ①.

82. Mr. Little says to the nurse, "I don't have much money. Will Medicare pay the hospital bill?" The nurse suggests that someone from social services visit Mr. Little to answer his questions and explain that

① Medicare pays the full cost of hospitalization for all persons over 65.

② Medicare is available only to those persons over 65 who are classified as financially underprivileged by the local welfare department.

③ persons over 65 who are receiving Social Security benefits are eligible for Medicare benefits.

④ persons over 65 who are hospitalized receive payments from Medicare automatically when hospitalization extends beyond two weeks.

The Patient Bill of Rights states that the client has a right to an explanation of his bill regardless of the source of payment. An explanation of Medicare benefits will put Mr. Little's mind at ease about how the bill can be paid. Correct answer ③.

Ms. Nancy Ker, 33 years old, is admitted to the hospital with a ruptured lumbar intervertebral disc. She is placed in pelvic traction. Ms. Kerr's prescriptions include heat applications and meperidine (Demerol) hydrochloride p.r.n. for pain.

83. Before applying heat to Ms. Kerr's lower back, it is essential to take which of these actions?

① Place a plastic protective covering on the skin before applying the source of heat.

② Apply a thin layer of petrolatum (Vaseline) on the skin before applying the source of heat.

③ Check the temperature of the source of heat.

④ Wrap the source of heat in a towel.

Although a heat source is usually wrapped in a towel, it is essential that the temperature of the heat source be checked prior to application. If the source is too hot a towel will not prevent a burn. Correct answer ③.

84. Ms. Kerr requires Demerol for pain. Before giving Ms. Kerr the Demerol, it would be most important for the nurse to take which of these actions?

① Check her pupillary responses.

② Count her respirations.

③ Determine her pulse deficit.

④ Assess her urinary output.

Demerol is a central nervous system depressant. Respiratory distress could occur after administration. Therefore Ms. Kerr's respiratory rate must be checked beforehand so that a baseline can be determined. If the rate is too low the drug should be withheld. Correct answer ②.

GO ON TO THE NEXT PAGE.

Ms. Kerr's response to medical therapy is unsatisfactory and she is scheduled for surgery.

85. Ms. Kerr asks the nurse if she may put makeup on before she goes to surgery. Understanding her responsibility to promote client safety, the nurse's best response would be,

① "The hospital regulations state that all makeup must be removed before you go to surgery, Ms. Kerr."

② "It depends upon the amount of makeup you use, Ms. Kerr."

③ "Makeup will interfere with seeing any changes in the color of your skin during surgery, Ms. Kerr."

④ "I'll check with the nurse in charge to see if it is all right for you to put your makeup on Ms. Kerr."

Accurate assessment of changes in skin color cannot be made if a client has makeup on. Established preoperative routines require removal of makeup in order to provide safe care. Correct answer ③.

Ms. Kerr has a laminectomy performed under general anesthesia. After several hours in the recovery room, Ms. Kerr is returned to her unit.

86. The logrolling technique is to be used to change Ms. Kerr's position. The purpose of using this technique for her is to

① increase the spaces between her vertebrae.

② provide adequate support for her extremities.

③ keep her from lying on her incision.

④ prevent strain on her surgical wound.

Logrolling allows for a position change without undue stress on the surgical wound or the back muscles. Although lying on the incision may be painful, it is not contraindicated. Correct answer ④.

87. Ms. Kerr's blood pressure has been stable at 130/80, and her pulse rate has been 80. Which of these vital signs would most clearly indicate the development of shock?

① Blood pressure 100/60; pulse 120.

② Blood pressure 120/80; pulse 74.

③ Blood pressure 140/100; pulse 100.

④ Blood pressure 150/90; pulse 60.

The development of shock is characterized by a dropping blood pressure and a rising pulse. Therefore a blood pressure of 100/60 and a pulse of 120 would signal shock in Ms. Kerr. Correct answer ①.

88. How should the nurse assist Ms. Kerr onto a bedpan?

① Tell her to flex her knees and raise her buttocks as the bedpan is put in place.

② Instruct her to use the overbed trapeze as a means of raising her hips so that the bedpan can be put in place.

③ Turn her onto her side, put the bedpan in place, and return her to a back-lying position on the bedpan.

④ Have her press down on the bed with her hands to raise her buttocks so that the bedpan can be put in place.

After a laminectomy, flexion of the spine should be avoided. The correct way for the nurse to arrange the bedpan is to turn Ms. Kerr to her side, put the bedpan in place, and return her to a back-lying position on the bedpan. Correct answer ③.

89. Ms. Kerr is ambulatory. On her fifth postoperative day, she complains of a sore area in her left calf. Which of these actions by the nurse would be best?

① Instruct Ms. Kerr to remain in bed and then report the symptom to the nurse in charge.

② Massage Ms. Kerr's left leg gently and than take her pedal pulse.

③ Have Ms. Kerr ambulate and then question her about the effect of the activity on her left leg.

④ Tell Ms. Kerr to move her left leg and then palpate it for other areas of soreness.

Both during and after a period of immobility, the client is at risk for the development of thrombophlebitis. The correct nursing intervention is to instruct Ms. Kerr to remain in bed and report the symptom to the charge nurse. Ambulation and massage could loosen the possible clot, causing an embolus. Correct answer ①.

Mr. Frank Anderman, 85 years old, has been in a skilled nursing facility for 10 months. He has generalized arteriosclerosis. Most of the patients are more than 80 years old.

90. The nurse caring for Mr. Anderman should anticipate that because of arteriosclerotic changes in the brain, he may experience confusion and disorientation during which of these times of day?

① Upon arising in the morning.

② When ambulating during the day.

③ When sitting alone in the afternoon.

④ Upon awakening during the night.

During the night it is dark; there is a lack of stimulation and a lack of personnel to establish a relationship between time and place. Mr. Anderman will be most confused when awakening in the middle of the night. Correct answer ④.

GO ON TO THE NEXT PAGE.

91. Mr. Anderman may have a diet as tolerated. The consistency of the diet served to him should be determined primarily by his

① age.
② ability to chew.
③ activity level.
④ food preferences.

To insure that Mr. Anderman's nutritional requirements are met, his ability to chew food must be assessed. Correct answer ②.

92. The normal physiologic changes occurring in old age result in a **decreased** nutritional need for

① vitamin B complex.
② calcium.
③ protein.
④ calories.

Overall nutritional needs of the elderly are essentially the same as other adults, except that their caloric needs diminish because they are simply maintaining a stable body structure. Correct answer ④.

93. It would be appropriate for the nurse to use three of the following measures to help patients like Mr. Anderman maintain normal bowel habits. Which one is the **exception**?

① Answering his request to go to the bathroom immediately.
② Having him drink a glass of water before each meal.
③ Establishing a daily schedule with him for having a bowel movement.
④ Massaging his abdomen after each bowel movement.

Notice that the question asks for the EXCEPTION. Answers ① through ③ are appropriate, but massaging Mr. Anderman's abdomen after each bowel movement is inappropriate and does not promote a therapeutic goal. Correct answer ④.

94. When the nurse is preparing Mr. Anderman for sleep, Mr. Anderman says, "I wake up at night because my feet get so cold. How can I keep them warm?" Which of these actions by the nurse would demonstrate the best judgment?

① Rub his feet briskly to improve the circulation.
② Place a light blanket over his feet.
③ Place his feet on a covered hot-water bottle.
④ Put a covered heating pad on his feet, with the dial turned to the lowest setting.

Placing a light blanket over Mr. Anderman's feet is the simplest and safest method of keeping them warm. Correct answer ②.

95. The skilled nursing facility where Mr. Anderman is a client decides to undertake a public campaign to promote safety for the elderly. The staff knows that the greatest number of accidents among the elderly result from

① falls.

② suicide.

③ vehicular collisions.

④ unintentional ingestion of poisons.

Because the aging process results in physical and mental instability, the elderly are prone to falling. Death may occur as a direct result of the fall or because of complications from injuries sustained. Correct answer ①.

Ms. Pamela Evan, 28 years old, is admitted to the hospital following a severe bleeding episode from a recurring peptic ulcer. Ms. Evan is scheduled for a subtotal gastrectomy. Her prescriptions include a cleansing enema.

---

96. Ms. Evan is to receive an enema of 1,000 ml. of solution. After receiving 100 ml. of the solution, Ms. Evan says to the nurse, "I can't hold any more. It's going to come out!"

Which of these actions would it be most appropriate for the nurse to take **first**?

① Remove the rectal tube, place Ms. Evan on the bedpan, and then attempt to give the remainder of the fluid later if she still needs it.

② Clamp the tubing, instruct Ms. Evan to take several deep breaths, and then wait a minute or two before releasing the clamp.

③ Inform Ms. Evan that additional fluid must be instilled and then lower the fluid container slightly.

④ Discontinue the procedure, place Ms. Evan on the bedpan, and then report the problem to the nurse in charge.

Clamping the tubing and instructing Ms. Evan to take deep breaths is the first appropriate intervention. This may help her hold the solution because it relaxes the abdominal muscles. Correct answer ②.

GO ON TO THE NEXT PAGE.

97. On the morning of surgery, the nurse is to care for Ms. Evan. As a basis for deciding when to give Ms. Evan her preoperative medication, the nurse should have which of these understandings?

① The preoperative medication should be given prior to morning care to allow for observation of Ms. Evan's reaction to the medication.

② The preoperative medication should be given prior to morning care to promote optimal relaxation in Ms. Evan.

③ Ms. Evan's morning care should be completed prior to giving her preoperative medication to prevent having to disturb her.

④ Ms. Evan's morning care should be completed prior to giving her preoperative medication because the medication will act rapidly in a person of her age.

The purpose of preoperative medication is to relax the client, alleviate anxiety, and permit smooth induction of anesthesia prior to surgery. Therefore, Ms. Evan should not be disturbed after the preoperative medication, and her morning care should be completed before the medication is given. Correct answer ③.

Ms. Evan has a subtotal gastrectomy. She is brought to the recovery room, with a nasogastric tube in place.

---

98. In the immediate postoperative period, which of these assessments of Ms. Evan should have priority?

① Presence of Babinski reflex.

② Patency of the airway.

③ Return of sensation to the legs.

④ Level of consciousness.

Patency of the airway is the highest priority in achieving pulmonary ventilation and preventing hypoxemia. Airway obstruction most frequently occurs as a result of the tongue, which is relaxed from anesthesia, falling back against the pharynx, or as a result of secretions or other fluids collecting in the trachea or bronchial tree. Correct answer ②.

After Ms. Evan reacts from anesthesia, she is brought back to her room. The nasogastric tube is attached to low, intermittent suction.

---

99. After Ms. Evan is transferred from the stretcher to her bed, the nurse takes her vital signs. Which of these actions should the nurse take next?

① Have her deep-breathe.

② Determine her need for medication to relieve pain.

③ Check her level of consciousness.

④ Inspect her dressing.

Inspecting Ms. Evan's dressing for bleeding should be the next action by the nurse. External bleeding, which could occur within the first 48 hours post surgery, would be detected by checking the dressing. Correct answer ④.

100. While Ms. Evan has the nasogastric tube in place, she is given mouth care frequently. What is a purpose of this measure?

① To maintain her ability to swallow.

② To prevent her from losing her gag reflex.

③ To keep the oral mucous membrane moist.

④ To stimulate peristalsis.

Mouth care will prevent dryness and discomfort for Ms. Evan by keeping the mucous membrane of the mouth moist. Correct answer ③.

101. While assisting Ms. Evan with her bath the day after her surgery, the nurse observes that the tape on one side of her dressing is no longer adhering to her skin.

Which of these actions would demonstrate the best judgment?

① Change the dressing.

② Retape the dressing.

③ Use an abdominal binder to hold the dressing in place.

④ Apply tincture of benzoin to the skin under the tape and press the tape firmly against the skin.

The nurse should retape the dressing while assisting with Ms. Evan's bath. Retaping the dressing holds it in place. Changing would not be appropriate because initial observation of the site requires assessment by the surgeon or registered nurse. Correct answer ②.

102. During the early postoperative period, Ms. Evan is encouraged to move her lower extremities frequently. The chief purpose of this measure is to prevent

① pressure sores.

② abdominal distention.

③ muscle atrophy.

④ venous stasis.

Venous stasis could lead to serious postoperative complications such as the formation of venous thrombosis. Exercising the legs helps to prevent this complication. Correct answer ④.

Mr. Roger Powell, 61 years old, is admitted to the hospital for observation following a car accident. The next day, it is determined that he has no physical injury resulting from the accident. It is learned that he was drunk while driving and that he has been drinking a quart of alcohol per day for the past 10 years. He is beginning to have delirium tremens. Blood studies and a diet high in protein and calories are prescribed for him.

GO ON TO THE NEXT PAGE.

103. The nurse who admits Mr. Powell records information about his health history. The nurse understands that persons who have a history of excessive drinking are most likely to manifest

① the development of a psychosis.

② physical problems that require medical evaluation.

③ a willingness to seek help.

④ an inability to follow simple instructions.

Laennec's cirrhosis results from chronic alcoholism and malnutrition. Clients will manifest the physical symptoms that accompany the gradual onset and extension of this chronic disease. Correct answer ②.

104. The nurse understands that Mr. Powell must be protected from injury if he develops delirium tremens. The **first** symptoms of delirium tremens are

① muscle rigidity and tension.

② agitation and anger.

③ restlessness and confusion.

④ abdominal distention and lethargy.

Delirium tremens are characterized by progressive disorientation about time and place. The client will be restless and confusion will become evident. As the condition advances, clients become agitated and combative. They may have auditory and visual hallucinations. Correct answer ③.

105. Mr. Powell's behavior during delirium tremens is unsettling to his wife, who expresses concern to the nurse. It would be best to convey to Ms. Powell which of these understandings about delirium tremens?

① It happens when alcoholism is combined with a psychiatric disorder.

② It is not serious and it usually disappears gradually within a few weeks.

③ It is not basically a serious disturbance, but the effects tend to be long-lasting.

④ It is frightening to observe, but it is usually temporary and subsides within a few days.

Delirium tremens, while potentially life-threatening, are temporary, with the majority of cases resolving within 2-4 days. The course of DT's may include thrashing, jerky movements, profuse sweating, and auditory and visual hallucinations which may frighten inexperienced observers. Correct answer ④.

106. As Mr. Powell recovers from delirium tremens, he repeatedly makes demands of the nurse. Which of these actions should the nurse take?

① Point out to Mr. Powell that his behavior suggests that he could now benefit from attending meetings of Alcoholics Anonymous.

② Tell Mr. Powell that he is demonstrating an abnormal degree of dependency.

③ Recognize that Mr. Powell may be troubled and take time to talk with him.

④ Let Mr. Powell know that his behavior is unreasonable and that the staff is trying to be tolerant.

Mr. Powell's inability to control his behavior during the episode of delirium tremens may have scared him and made him fearful of losing control again. His repeated demands are a method to control his environment. The nurse can be most therapeutic by spending time with Mr. Powell and talking to him about his concerns. Correct answer ③.

107. The nurse reads Mr. Powell's medical record to plan for his specific nursing care. His physician has prescribed hemoglobin and hematocrit determinations to ascertain the presence of

① leukemia.

② uremia.

③ erythema.

④ anemia.

Hemoglobin is the oxygen carrying pigment of the red blood cells. Hematocrit measures the relative volume of cells and plasma in the blood. Both are tests for anemia. Clients with anemia require special nursing considerations relating to fatigue, weakness, and nutrition. Correct answer ④.

108. In view of the prescribed diet high in protein and calories for Mr. Powell, which of these menus would be best for him?

① Bacon, lettuce, and tomato sandwich, fruited gelatin dessert with whipped topping, and cola drink.

② Hot roast beef sandwich with gravy, mashed potatoes, green beans, chocolate pudding, and fruit punch.

③ Beefburger patty, cucumber salad, cooked carrots, apple, and orange juice.

④ Macaroni with tomato sauce, spinach, pear, and milk.

The roast beef sandwich and chocolate pudding provide a high amount of protein, and more calories than, for example, the third menu which contains protein in the beefburger, but lower calories in the rest of the meal. Correct answer ②.

GO ON TO THE NEXT PAGE.

Ms. Hilda Turner, 54 years old, is admitted to the hospital. She has a history of ulcerative colitis and she is scheduled to have an abdominal perineal resection.

109. On the evening prior to surgery, the nurse is teaching Ms. Turner coughing and breathing exercises. She says, "Stop treating me like a child. I wouldn't be here now if I hadn't learned to breathe a long time ago."

Which of these responses should the nurse make?

① "You know the reason for doing this."

② "You feel I'm talking down to you."

③ "You're overreacting."

④ "No one else has had that complaint."

The nurse should keep communication open, despite the fact that Ms. Turner is being difficult. By responding with, "You think I'm talking down to you," the nurse shows respect for Ms. Turner's feelings and allows her to calm down. The other responses are unnecessarily argumentative. Correct answer ②.

110. On the morning of her surgery, Ms. Turner has a nasogastric tube inserted. The purpose of this tube for Ms. Turner is to

① remove gas and fluids from the stomach.

② promote peristalsis in the large intestine.

③ prevent accumulation of fecal matter in the large intestine.

④ provide a means of administering nourishment postoperatively.

In order to remove gas and fluids from the stomach, the physician will usually prescribe gastric decompression by use of a nasogastric tube. This procedure prevents nausea, vomiting and distention that could occur after surgery due to decreased peristalsis. Correct answer ①.

Ms. Turner has surgery as scheduled and an ileostomy is performed. She has an ileostomy bag in place. Her condition is good when she is returned to the unit.

111. In Ms. Turner's early postoperative care, it would be most important to take measures to

① improve her respiratory function.

② increase her nutritional intake.

③ establish a routine pattern for urine elimination.

④ promote expulsion of flatus.

It would be most important to have Ms. Turner breathe deeply and cough in order to prevent postoperative complications such as atelectasis and pneumonia. Improving respiratory function is the most important goal of postoperative care. Correct answer ①.

112. When changing Ms. Turner's ileostomy bag, it is especially important that the nurse take which of these measures?

① Refraining from showing distaste.

② Maintaining strict surgical asepsis.

③ Explaining the details of the procedure.

④ Wiping the stoma with a mild antiseptic.

Most ileostomy clients worry about odor control and bowel excretion. They will take the attitude of the nurse as an example of the way other people will react. By not showing distaste when changing Ms. Turner's ileostomy bag, the nurse is teaching Ms. Turner to be unembarrassed about caring for her ileostomy. Correct answer ①.

113. Arrangements are made for Ms. Turner to be visited by a woman who has adjusted well to her ileostomy. Which of these actions by the nurse would probably promote the effectiveness of the visit?

① Remain in the room while the interview is in progress.

② Return to the room periodically to answer any questions that may arise.

③ Provide a quiet, private setting for the visit.

④ Maintain a detached manner until the visit is over.

The ostomy visitor will usually check with the nurse about any specifics to be discussed. Then the visitor should be introduced to the client. After the introduction, the client and visitor should be allowed a quiet, private visit. Correct answer ③.

114. On several occasions, Ms. Turner is observed picking at the food on her tray and eating very little. When questioned by the nurse, Ms. Turner says that she doesn't feel like eating.

Which of these actions by the nurse would be best?

① Ask Ms. Turner if she would like her husband to bring in food from home.

② Explain to Ms. Turner the importance of good nutrition to her recovery.

③ Tell Ms. Turner that her refusal to eat will have to be reported to both the nurse in charge and the physician.

④ Find out if Ms. Turner likes the meals she has been served.

The simplest explanation for Ms. Turner's lack of appetite is that the meals don't appeal to her. The nurse should ask if she likes her food before assuming the problem is bigger than it really is. Correct answer ④.

GO ON TO THE NEXT PAGE.

Mr. Spencer Otto, 22 years old, is brought to the emergency room following a motorcycle accident. He has a head injury and is semicomatose.

115. When Mr. Otto arrives in the emergency room, the initial action that should be taken is to

① check his vital signs.

② assess the extent of his injury.

③ determine the patency of his airway.

④ institute measures to prevent infection.

In an emergency situation, the first action taken must be the determination and maintenance of a patent airway. Without adequate respiratory function, all other measures are futile. Correct answer ③.

Mr. Otto is admitted to the hospital. His prescriptions include a spinal tap.

116. When Mr. Otto is brought to the unit, he should be placed in which of these positions?

① Head elevated slightly and turned to the side.

② Supine, with hyperextension of the neck.

③ Legs elevated and head on a small, firm pillow.

④ Trendelenburg.

A comatose client may aspirate stomach contents. Elevating the head will decrease the possibility of aspiration. Turning the client's head to the side will promote drainage of any vomitus. Correct answer ①.

117. During the spinal tap, the primary function of the nurse is to

① explain to the client the steps of the procedure as they occur.

② help the client to remain motionless.

③ prepare the labels for the fluid specimens.

④ apply pressure to the insertion site as the needle is being removed.

To insure a safe spinal tap, the client must remain perfectly still. The primary function of the nurse is to help the patient remain motionless throughout the procedure. (Labels can be prepared prior to the procedure). Correct answer ②.

118. One morning when the nurse enters Mr. Otto's room, he is beginning to have a seizure. Which of these actions should the nurse take?

① Suction his oropharynx.

② Restrain his extremities.

③ Help him to turn onto his abdomen.

④ Observe the progress of his tremors.

Accurate observation, description and documentation of the tremors and their progression are necessary to classify the type of seizure. Restriction of movement may result in broken bones. Correct answer ④.

119. It will be important to make three of the following observations of Mr. Otto while he is having the seizure. Which one would be **unnecessary**?

① The rate and volume of his pulse.

② The presence or absence of incontinence.

③ The length of his seizure.

④ The parts of his body affected by the seizure.

Body parts involved during a seizure can indicate the site of seizure origin in the brain. Ability to maintain control of voluntary muscles, such as the bladder, also indicates site of origin. The length of the seizure is important information. Pulse rate and volume are NOT important indicators of seizure activity, and therefore the right answer. Correct answer ①.

120. The early onset of increased intracranial pressure would be indicated by which of these signs?

① Oliguria.

② Pallor.

③ Widening pulse pressure.

④ Sudden decrease in body temperature.

Increased intracranial pressure is demonstrated by the following symptoms: headache, vomiting, papilledema, respiratory and skin changes. A widening of the pulse pressure (the difference between the systolic and diastolic blood pressure) is a reaction to ischemia of the vasomotor center. Correct answer ③.

THIS IS THE END OF PART I

The National Council Licensure Examination for Practical Nurses

PART II

You will be allowed 2 hours
to complete this part of the examination.

Please begin.

GENERAL INSTRUCTIONS: Proceed exactly as you did in answering the questions in Part I of this examination.

The first section of the test consists of questions relating to medical-surgical nursing.

Ms. Velma Quinn, 42 years old, goes to her physician because she has not been feeling well. A tentative diagnosis of hyperthyroidism is made, and diagnostic tests are to be done in the ambulatory care center.

1. The nurse in the ambulatory care unit asks Ms. Quinn about her symptoms. The nurse knows that Ms. Quinn has an increased secretion of thyroxin and anticipates her complaints of

① loss of appetite and abnormal pigmentation.

② insomnia and palpitations.

③ polyuria and excessive thirst.

④ diaphoresis and disorientation.

Increased secretion of thyroxin results in an increased metabolic rate which produces insomnia and palpitations. Correct answer ②.

2. The nurse is asked to make out the laboratory slips after the physician writes Ms. Quinn's prescriptions. To confirm a diagnosis of hyperthyroidism, the physician will have prescribed which of these tests?

① Protein-bound iodine and radioactive T-3 red cell uptake.

② Flat plate of the chest and brain scan.

③ Thyroid scan and hemoglobin.

④ Electroencephalogram and electrocardiogram.

Protein bound iodine (PBI) and radioactive T-3 red cell uptake are tests run on a venous blood sample to determine thyroid function. Correct answer ①.

3. The nurse asks Ms. Quinn if she has any other symptoms, knowing that because of Ms. Quinn's enlarged thyroid gland she may be experiencing

① a feeling of pressure on the trachea.

② a sensation of tickling in the oropharynx.

③ an impairment of hearing.

④ pain over the sternum.

The thyroid gland is located in the neck in front of the trachea. Correct answer ①.

A diagnosis of hyperthyroidism is confirmed.

4. Carbohydrates are very important in Ms. Quinn's diet at this time because they

① are easily stored by the body.

② are easy to digest.

③ provide amino acids.

④ provide a readily available source of energy.

Due to the hyperthyroidism, Ms. Quinn has an increased metabolic demand and needs the readily available energy provided by carbohydrates. Carbohydrate consumption also prevents liver damage from the depletion of glycogen. Correct answer ④.

5. In the treatment of clients with hyperthyroidism, which of these medications is likely to be prescribed to decrease the activity of the thyroid gland?

① Diazepam (Valium).

② Liothyronine sodium (Cytomel).

③ Prednisone.

④ Propylthiouracil.

Only anti-thyroid drugs can decrease thyroid gland activity. Muscle relaxants and steroids have no effect on thyroid function. Synthetic thyroid hormones (Cytomel) would increase thyroid gland activity. Propylthiouracil interferes with formation of thyroxin, thereby decreasing thyroid gland activity. Correct answer ④.

Ms. Quinn is admitted to the hospital and she has a subtotal thyroidectomy. She is returned to the surgical unit after a short stay in the recovery room. She is receiving fluids intravenously.

6. When Ms. Quinn has completely reacted from anesthesia and her vital signs are stable, which of these positions would be best for her?

① Prone.

② Semi-Fowler's.

③ Trendelenburg.

④ Supine.

The Semi-Fowler's position, with the head of the bed elevated and the knees also elevated, is the best way to maintain a patent airway, decrease the possibility of hemorrhage and rupture of sutures, and maintain client comfort. Correct answer ②.

7. Which of the following information about Ms. Quinn's intravenous therapy will it be essential for the licensed practical nurse to have?

① The specific purpose of giving Ms. Quinn intravenous fluids.

② The total amount of intravenous fluid in the bottle.

③ The desired rate of flow of the intravenous infusion.

④ The amount of urine Ms. Quinn can be expected to excrete in relation to the amount of fluid that she is receiving intravenously.

Administration of intravenous fluids can produce unwanted side effects if the fluid is infused too quickly or too slowly. Therefore, the nurse must know the desired flow rate for each intravenous infusion. Correct answer ③.

Mr. Thomas Hale, 33 years old, is admitted to the hospital. Mr. Hale has acute pyelonephritis. Prescriptions for Mr. Hale include bed rest, fluids ad lib., blood chemistry tests, and urine for culture and sensitivity testing.

---

8. Mr. Hale is to be on bed rest for which of these purposes?

① To prevent respiratory infection by reducing his contact with other persons.

② To insure safety while his body has increased toxins in the bloodstream.

③ To assist his body's defenses in combating infection.

④ To control ascending urinary infection by maintaining him in a horizontal position.

Bed rest will conserve energy and allow the body to use its resources to combat infection. Correct answer ③.

9. To obtain a urine specimen for culture from Mr. Hale, which of these actions is essential?

① Encourage him to drink fluids before his urine is collected.

② Place a preservative in the receptable in which his urine is to be collected.

③ Collect the first urine that he voids in the morning.

④ Use aseptic technique in collecting his urine.

Use of aseptic technique in collecting Mr. Hale's urine lowers the possibility of contamination with organisms from other sources. Culturing the specimen requires growing the organism and identifying antibiotics to which it is sensitive. Correct answer ④.

10. Mr. Hale's fluid intake and output are being measured. At breakfast Mr. Hale drank 6 ounces of coffee and 4½ ounces of orange juice. How many milliliters of fluid did he drink?

① 135
② 205
③ 245
④ 315

There are 30 milliliters in one ounce of fluid. Therefore:

$$\begin{array}{r} 30 \text{ milliliters} \\ \times 6 \text{ ounces} \\ \hline 180 \text{ millileters} \end{array} \qquad \begin{array}{r} 30 \text{ ml.} \\ \times 4.5 \text{ ounces} \\ \hline 150 \\ 120 \\ \hline 135.0 \text{ ml} \end{array}$$

$$\begin{array}{r} 180 \text{ ml. coffee} \\ + 135 \text{ ml. juice} \\ \hline 315 \text{ ml. fluid} \end{array}$$

Mr. Hale drank 315 ml. fluid. Correct answer ④.

Ms. Ida Young, 65 years old, complains of coldness, numbness, and tingling sensations in her lower extremities. There is an area of ulceration on her left ankle. After an examination by her physician, Ms. Young is admitted to the hospital with peripheral vascular disease and diabetes mellitus. Her admission prescriptions include bed rest and warm, moist packs to the ulcer site.

---

11. The nurse who is admitting Ms. Young should make certain that which of these items is added to her bed?

① Bed board.
② Bed cradle.
③ Shock blocks.
④ Trapeze bar.

The client is showing symptoms of impaired circulation. Nothing should be done to further impede her circulation, and the weight of the bed linen could be a source of pressure. Correct answer ②.

12. In applying the moist packs to Ms. Young's ankle, the nurse should use aseptic technique for which of these purposes?

① To destroy bacteria on the skin.
② To inhibit the growth of pathogens.
③ To prevent the introduction of additional microorganisms.
④ To minimize the risk of spreading infection to others.

Sterile technique reduces the risk of introducing additional microorganisms to the skin. Clients with diabetes heal poorly and their treatment should include prevention of infection. Correct answer ③.

GO ON TO THE NEXT PAGE.

13. The nurse should observe most closely which of these properties of the moist packs that are used for Ms. Young?

① Temperature.

② Size.

③ Type of solution.

④ Type of dressing.

One of Ms. Young's symptoms is numbness. She might not be able to feel intense heat and could be burned. Correct answer ①.

14. Knowing that Ms. Young's diabetes mellitus has not been controlled, the nurse is aware that Ms. Young may complain about which of these symptoms?

① Anorexia and constipation.

② Tremors and irritability.

③ Excessive thirst and voiding of large amounts of urine.

④ Excessive weight gain and excessive perspiration.

Polydipsia and polyuria are symptoms of diabetes mellitus. Correct answer ③.

The physician prescribes a 1,500-calorie diabetic diet for Ms. Young and 30 units of isophane (NPH) insulin U-100 daily.

---

15. Ms. Young is to have a midafternoon snack of milk and crackers. The purpose of this measure for her is to

① improve nutrition.

② improve carbohydrate metabolism.

③ prevent an insulin reaction.

④ prevent diabetic coma.

NPH insulin is an intermediate acting insulin with a peak action of 6 to 8 hours. During peak action time, maximum insulin effect is expected to occur. To prevent an insulin reaction, proper food supplements must be given. Correct answer ③.

16. Insulin is administered in the treatment of diabetes mellitus in order to

① stimulate the secretion of insulin in the body.

② meet the metabolic need for insulin.

③ depress the activity of beta cells of the pancreas.

④ suppress the production of glycogen.

The purpose of administering insulin is to replace a deficiency in the client's metabolic system. Insulin lowers the blood glucose level and enables the body to metabolize carbohydrates. Correct answer ②.

17. While the nurse is administering an insulin injection, Ms. Young asks, "Why can't you give me a pill?" The nurse's response should be based on which of the following information?

① Oral drugs used for diabetes mellitus are not insulin.

② Oral drugs used for diabetes mellitus act more rapidly than insulin by injection.

③ The oral drug is a natural product whereas insulin for injection is a synthetic product.

④ There is no difference between the oral drug and insulin for injection.

Oral hypoglycemic drugs are classified as sulfonylureas; they are not insulin. Correct answer ①.

18. Ms. Young is taught to test her urine for sugar four times a day. At which of these times should the test be done?

① Upon arising in the morning and after meals.

② Before meals and at bedtime.

③ Every six hours.

④ Between meals, at 8 p.m., and at midnight.

Urine testing should be done before meals and at bedtime in order to evaluate more accurately the client's response to treatment and whether adjustments are needed. Correct answer ②.

19. Ms. Young is being observed for symptoms of insulin reaction. Early symptoms of insulin reaction include

① abdominal pain and nausea.

② dyspnea and pallor.

③ flushing of the skin and headache.

④ perspiration and a trembling sensation.

Too much insulin in the bloodstream in relation to glucose can cause the person with diabetes to experience an insulin reaction. Symptoms that signal onset of insulin reaction are sweating, weakness, dizziness, trembling sensation or irritable behavior. The client must drink or eat something to raise blood sugar. Correct answer ④.

20. The nurse is encouraging Ms. Young to take better care of herself. One day the nurse enters the room just as Ms. Young is lighting a cigarette. Ms. Young says, "My doctor has advised me to stop smoking."

The nurse's response should be based on which of these understandings about smoking cigarettes?

① Nicotine in cigarettes is a vasoconstrictor.

② Cigarettes are carcinogenic.

③ Smoking is a bronchial irritant.

④ Smoking causes arteriosclerosis.

Nicotine is a vasoconstrictor and contributes to progressive peripheral vascular disease. Correct answer ①.

GO ON TO THE NEXT PAGE.

21. To take care of her feet properly, Ms. Young needs to know that it is necessary to

① soak her feet daily in water containing magnesium sulfate (Epsom salt).

② cut her toenails straight across.

③ remove calluses as soon as possible.

④ apply lotion liberally, especially between the toes.

To avoid injury to the toes, Ms. Young should be taught to cut her toe nails straight across. Even slight abrasions or scratches can lead to serious problems for clients with diabetes because of their impaired circulation. Correct answer ②.

22. Before Ms. Young's teaching program is completed, it will be important for her to have which of these understandings about managing her diabetes mellitus?

① Sugar-free urine is the best indicator of the control of diabetes mellitus.

② Diabetes mellitus can be cured if the measures prescribed by the physician are followed closely.

③ Self-regulation of insulin dosage is the primary goal.

④ Symptoms of any illness warrant the immediate notification of the physician.

The client with diabetes should understand that any illness may cause an alteration in the diabetic state, and should be brought to the attention of the physician. Following physician orders and regular urine testing are necessary. Correct answer ④.

23. Ms. Young should be instructed to recognize the common early symptoms of diabetic acidosis, which include

① thirst and drowsiness.

② cold, clammy skin and anxiety.

③ slow pulse and increased blood pressure.

④ bulging of the eyeballs and dark amber urine.

The onset of diabetic acidosis is gradual, the specific cause being lack of insulin and eventual accumulation of glucose and waste products from excessive fat and protein metabolism. Ms. Young should be instructed to recognize thirst and drowsiness as symptoms of diabetic acidosis. Correct answer ①.

Mr. Owen David, a 19-year-old college student, has difficulty in swallowing, an elevated temperature, and chronic fatigue. He is admitted to the hospital. The results of diagnostic tests reveal that Mr. David has infectious mononucleosis with liver involvement. His prescriptions include a diet high in calories, protein, and vitamins.

24. Because of the liver involvement, Mr. David should be expected to have which of these symptoms?

① Constipation.

② Excessive thirst.

③ Anorexia.

④ Hematuria.

Anorexia is a common problem in clients with liver involvement because the liver is important in metabolism. Correct answer ③.

25. Mr. David develops stomatitis. His mouth care should include which of these measures?

① Rinsing his mouth with an astringent mouthwash.

② Cleansing his mouth frequently with a nonabrasive material.

③ Applying mineral oil to his irritated mucosa.

④ Coating his oral cavity with an antiseptic solution.

Cleansing Mr. David's mouth with a nonabrasive solution is the safest method of mouth care because the mucus is susceptible to trauma. Correct answer ②.

26. Which of these behaviors is characteristic of a normal adolescent of Mr. David's age?

① Conforming to adult standards.

② Worrying about athletic ability.

③ Having conflicts between dependence and independence.

④ Having definite vocational goals.

Having conflicts between dependence and independence is a normal characteristic of adolescents moving toward adulthood. These conflicts represent a search for identity. Correct answer ③.

The next section of the test consists of individual questions relating to medical-surgical nursing.

---

27. A female client who is terminally ill is working through her feelings about dying. The degree to which the nurse can give support to this client will be determined by which of these factors?

① The ability of the nurse to adhere to hospital policy regarding care of dying clients.

② The physician's willingness to prepare the client for death.

③ The age of the client and the frequency with which the nurse has to give support to the dying.

④ The nurse's feelings about death and the quality of the nurse's relationship with the client.

Ability to provide support to a dying client depends on the nurse's own feelings and beliefs about death and dying. A client is more likely to discuss these personal issues with the nurses who have developed a beneficial, therapeutic relationship with her. Correct answer ④.

GO ON TO THE NEXT PAGE.

28. Which of these foods are good sources of vitamin A?

① Roast beef and bacon.

② Corn and yellow beans.

③ Orange juice and bananas.

④ Carrots and sweet potatoes.

The ultimate source of all vitamin A is plants, especially those with carotene. Carrots and sweet potatoes are the only foods listed that have carotene. Correct answer ④.

29. The urine of a client with high levels of bilirubin in the blood can be expected to be which of these colors?

① Clear yellow.

② Dark amber.

③ Red.

④ Green.

Many substances and medications can discolor a client's urine. High levels of bilirubin in the blood will color urine a dark amber. Correct answer ②.

30. A client who has just been diagnosed as having glaucoma says to the nurse, "I hope the treatment will improve my vision." The nurse's reply should be based on which of these understandings of the prognosis of glaucoma?

① Blindness will eventually develop, but treatment will delay it.

② Vision already lost cannot be restored, and continuous treatment is necessary to prevent further visual loss.

③ Special eyeglasses will correct the visual impairment that occurs, but the lenses must be changed frequently.

④ Surgery can restore lost vision.

Glaucoma is caused by changes in the anterior chamber of the eye, which prevent normal outflow of aqueous humor and cause increased intraocular pressure. Continued pressure causes damage to the optic nerve and visual loss. If the disease is not treated blindness will occur. Correct answer ②.

31. Which of these measures is essential in the care of a client who is in a coma?

① Checking the client's blood pressure every 2 hours.

② Maintaining the client in a semi-Fowler's position.

③ Turning the client from side to side at regular intervals.

④ Addressing the client in a loud tone.

A comatose client, unable to move independently, can develop many side effects including pneumonia and decubitus ulcers. Turning the client from side to side at regular intervals will distribute the pressure among many points, decreasing the possibility of decubitus ulcer formation. These position changes will also help drain secretions from the lungs. Correct answer ③.

32. During the first few hours after having a liver biopsy, a client should be observed for which of these complications?

① Gastric irritation.

② Infection.

③ Allergic reactions.

④ Hemorrhage.

A liver biopsy is an invasive technique involving the use of a special biopsy needle. Hemorrhage is a complication that will appear in the first hours following this procedure. Correct answer ④.

33. Colostomy irrigations have been prescribed for a client. Which of these understandings is essential for safe performance of a colostomy irrigation?

① Absorption of the irrigating fluid in the intestinal tract will be affected by the client's position.

② The pressure of the irrigating fluid in the intestinal tract will be determined by the height at which the fluid container is held.

③ The irrigating fluid dilates the blood vessels of the intestinal tract.

④ Manipulation of the irrigation catheter results in muscle spasm of the intestinal tract.

Introduction of colostomy irrigation fluid under high pressure can lead to perforation of the intestines. Since the irrigation fluid is introduced using a simple pressure principle, the nurse should understand that the pressure of the fluid will be increased the higher the fluid container is held above the client. Pressure can be reduced by placing the irrigation fluid container near the level of the client's abdomen. Correct answer ②.

The next section of the test consists of questions relating to maternity nursing.

Ms. Ann Lasher, 20 years old, attends the antepartal clinic. The physician examines Ms. Lasher and finds her to be about 3 months pregnant.

---

34. Ms. Lasher's physician has written a prescription for vitamins. The nurse gives Ms. Lasher the prescription and also tells her that vegetables are a good source of vitamins and minerals particularly if

① eaten raw.

② stored in the refrigerator.

③ cooked in unsalted water.

④ boiled in a covered pot.

Fresh, raw produce will contain all its natural nutrients. Cooking destroys some vitamins and minerals. Correct answer ①.

35. Ms. Lasher states that she never drinks milk. The nurse asks if she is allergic to milk. Ms. Lasher answers, "No, I just don't like the taste of it."

Which response by the nurse would be best?

① Ask Ms. Lasher what foods she likes that contain milk.

② Ask Ms. Lasher if she understands why milk is important for the development of her baby.

③ Suggest that Ms. Lasher substitute one whole egg for every glass of milk that she omits from her diet.

④ Suggest that Ms. Lasher talk with her physician about taking calcium tablets as a substitute for milk.

Milk is an important source of the whole proteins and vitamin D essential for fetal development and maternal health. It is necessary to determine a food allergy to milk or milk products and then recommend alternate sources of the nutrients contained in milk. Correct answer ①.

36. During Ms. Lasher's clinic visit when she is 4 months pregnant, which of these procedures will be carried out for her?

① Vaginal smear and pelvic measurements.

② Vaginal examination and Rh factor determination.

③ Blood test for syphilis and rectal examination.

④ Blood pressure determination and weighing.

Monitoring Ms. Lasher's blood pressure and weight is part of each prenatal visit. During the second trimester of pregnancy, signs of preeclampsia may appear. These include elevated blood pressure and edema which may be evidenced by sudden weight gain. Correct answer ④.

37. Ms. Lasher states that she works out 3 or 4 times a week and asks how much exercise she can safely do while she is pregnant. The nurse responds based on the understanding that

① activities that require stretching and bending should be avoided.

② usual activities should be continued in moderation.

③ emphasis should be given to active participation in outdoor activities.

④ each new activity should be preceded by a short period of rest.

Moderation is the key to all activity during pregnancy. Correct answer ②.

Ms. Lasher's pregnancy progresses normally. She is admitted to the hospital at term and has a normal spontaneous delivery of a girl. Ms. Lasher plans to breast feed her infant.

38. When Ms. Lasher is 6 hours postpartum, she is placed on a bedpan to void. After trying for a period of time, Mrs. Lasher states that she is unable to void. Her bladder is distended.

Which of these measures would it be best for the nurse to use to help Ms. Lasher to void?

① Pour warm water over her vulva.

② Apply gentle manual pressure over her bladder.

③ Encourage her to drink fluids freely.

④ Explain to her that she will have to be catheterized if she does not void.

Pouring warm water over the vulva is a helpful nursing measure which may stimulate the client to void. The warm temperature may help relax the meatus and the sensation of running water encourages urine release. Correct answer ①.

39. When Baby Girl Lasher is brought to Ms. Lasher for the first breast feeding, Ms. Lasher asks the nurse, "How much of the nipple should the baby be given?"

Which of these replies is it correct for the nurse to give Ms. Lasher?

① "The baby should have the nipple and some of the dark area around the nipple well into her mouth."

② "Since she's had some water from a bottle in the nursery, she has already learned the amount of nipple she needs to nurse adequately."

③ "Babies' mouths are of different sizes, and the baby will take the correct amount of nipple for her."

④ "Babies nurse best when only the nipple is in the mouth."

Placing the areola (dark area) as well as the nipple in the baby's mouth aids in adequately compressing the milk ducts underneath the pigmented skin. Also, this placement decreases stress on the nipple leading to cracks and soreness. Correct answer ①.

40. On Ms. Lasher's third postpartum day, the nurse finds her crying. When asked what seems to be wrong, Ms. Lasher says, "I really don't know. I have so much to be grateful for—a healthy baby, a good husband—I really should be happy."

Which of these actions by the nurse would demonstrate the best judgment in this situation?

① Provide privacy for Ms. Lasher.

② Ask Ms. Lasher if her relationship with her husband will permit her to discuss her feelings with him.

③ Explain to Ms. Lasher that her reaction is an unusual one.

④ Remain with Ms. Lasher for a while.

By remaining with Ms. Lasher the nurse demonstrates empathy and concern for the client. Her supportive presence may encourage Ms. Lasher to verbalize further and better understand her feelings. Correct answer ④.

GO ON TO THE NEXT PAGE.

41. Because Ms. Lasher is breast feeding her baby, in which of these ways is the diet recommended for her likely to **differ** from that recommended for a mother who is not nursing?

① It is lower in roughage and higher in carbohydrates.

② It is lower in sodium and higher in iron.

③ It is higher in calcium and protein.

④ It is higher in fat and cellulose.

During lactation a mother needs additional calcium and protein in her diet. Milk production places great demand on the mother's resources of both these substances. Correct answer ③.

Ms. Dora Stone, 31 years old, comes to the antepartal clinic because she has missed 2 menstrual periods. She is found to be about 10 weeks pregnant. This is Ms. Stone's third pregnancy. The Stones have 2 children.

---

42. Ms. Stone has been advised by the physician to increase her intake of iron. Which of these sandwiches, as ordinarily prepared, is **highest** in iron?

① Egg salad.

② Peanut butter.

③ Cream cheese and jelly.

④ Lettuce and tomato.

Eggs contain approximately 1.2 mg. of iron per egg; none of the foods in the other answers contain an appreciable amount of iron. Correct answer ①.

Ms. Stone attends the clinic when she is 8 months pregnant.

---

43. Three of the following symptoms are common at this stage of pregnancy. Which one is the **exception**?

① Frequent urination.

② Nausea and vomiting.

③ Edema of the ankles.

④ Dyspnea when lying flat in bed.

When nausea and vomiting occur they tend to be symptoms experienced in the first trimester of pregnancy. Ms. Stone is 8 months pregnant, and nausea and vomiting would be unusual at this stage of pregnancy. Correct answer ②.

44. Ms. Stone says to the nurse, "Sometimes I think about what would happen if I died during childbirth." Which of these approaches by the nurse would be best?

① Explain to her that such thoughts are common at her stage of pregnancy.

② Tell her that maternal deaths are extremely rare.

③ Find out what prompted these feelings in her.

④ Ask her if she has discussed these feelings with her husband.

The nurse needs to find the underlying reason for Ms. Stone's expression of fear about childbirth. Three of the responses dismiss Ms. Stone's fears and cut off any further discussion. The third response allows the nurse to find out more about Ms. Stone's anxiety. Correct answer ③.

At term Ms. Stone is admitted to the hospital in active labor. Ms. Stone's labor is being electronically monitored.

45. Ms. Stone asks what is happening as the nurse summons the charge nurse to the labor room.

The nurse's action would be in response to which of the following symptoms?

① A decrease in the fetal heart rate from 144 to 132 during a contraction.

② A decrease in the interval between contractions from 6 to 7 minutes to 4 to 5 minutes.

③ A sudden increase in the amount of blood in the vaginal show.

④ An increase in blood pressure from 120/76 to 132/80 at the beginning of a contraction.

The nurse recognizes that an increase of blood in the vaginal show might be a symptom of a placenta previa or abruptio placentae. She calls the nurse in charge because she legally is working under the direction of a registered nurse. Her response to Ms. Stone will be within the framework of the client's right to know. Correct answer ③.

Ms. Stone's labor progresses normally. She delivers a boy.

46. A few hours after Ms. Stone's delivery, the nurse notes that Ms. Stone has saturated two perineal pads with blood within a 20-minute period. Which of these actions should the nurse take **first**?

① Check the consistency of Ms. Stone's uterine fundus.

② Encourage Ms. Stone to void.

③ Take Ms. Stone's blood pressure.

④ Notify the nurse in charge.

By assessing the consistency of Ms. Stone's uterine fundus the nurse may be able to take steps to control the bleeding. If the fundus is not well contracted, fundal massage may stimulate contraction and reduce bleeding. The nurse may then implement other actions. While all the answers are correct, the best action to take is ①. Correct answer ①.

Ms. Stone is transferred to the postpartum unit.

47. Ms. Stone says to the nurse, "I guess I really want some help. I don't need any more children. Three are enough." Which of these approaches by the nurse would be best **first**?

① Find out what Ms. Stone knows about the availability of family planning services.

② Ask Ms. Stone if her husband is interested in conception control.

③ Discuss with Ms. Stone the effectiveness of various contraceptive methods.

④ Commend Ms. Stone for her determination to limit her family size.

Before proceeding with health teaching it is always best to assess the client's level of knowledge on the subject. By finding out what Ms. Stone knows about available services, the nurse can assist her in making a decision about further counseling. Correct answer ①.

Ms. Liane Wilson, 35 years old, has 6 children, aged 1, 2, 3, 5, 7, and 9 years. Ms. Wilson is visiting the physician because she has not menstruated for several months.

48. In the waiting room, Ms. Wilson says to another client, "Here I am again. I kind of hope that I'm not pregnant." When the nurse is helping Ms. Wilson to prepare for her examination, the nurse says to Ms. Wilson, "I overheard your comments to the other patient in the waiting room."

Which of these additional remarks by the nurse would be most appropriate to follow this initial comment?

① "You may feel negative about another pregnancy now. These feelings are bound to change."

② "It's healthy to express your feelings. Let's talk about them."

③ "You ought to discuss these feelings with the doctor, since they may affect the outcome of your pregnancy."

④ "The doctor may advise you to seek professional counseling. Such feelings often precede emotional problems in the postpartum period."

By giving the client the cue that discussion of feelings is healthy, the nurse encourages her to talk about her reaction to her pregnancy. It also gives recognition to the importance of these feelings. Correct answer ②.

Ms. Wilson is about 3 months pregnant.

49. Ms. Wilson's physician directs the nurse to assist with a test to confirm Ms. Wilson's presumed pregnancy. Which of the following will the nurse be asked to do?

① Bring a fetoscope with which to listen for fetal heart tones.

② Collect a urine specimen to test for chorionic gonadotropin.

③ Prepare Ms. Stone for an x-ray to show the fetal skeleton.

④ Collect a blood sample to check for the presence of pituotrin.

To confirm a diagnosis of pregnancy, the physician would order a urine test. Chorionic gonadotropin is present in a pregnant woman's urine ten days after the first missed period. Correct answer ②.

50. As she is leaving the physician's office, Ms. Wilson says to the nurse, "The doctor wants me to keep all of my appointments and follow his directions carefully. After 6 babies I can take care of myself." The nurse encourages Ms. Wilson to follow the physician's instructions, knowing that

① premature labor is a common occurrence in women such as Ms. Wilson who are extremely active and over 25 years of age.

② fetal anoxia results from placental aging, which is common in women of Ms. Wilson's age group.

③ multigravidas are especially susceptible to infectious diseases.

④ grand multiparas have a higher incidence of complications.

The nurse understands that women over 35 and women who have had 5 or more pregnancies are considered high risk mothers. Correct answer ④.

GO ON TO THE NEXT PAGE.

At term Ms. Wilson is admitted to the hospital and delivers a 9-lb., 4-oz. (4,196-gm.) boy. Ms. Wilson is planning to breast feed her baby.

51. At 5 minutes of life, Baby Boy Wilson's Apgar score is 9. Which of these findings is **NOT** present in babies with such a score?

① Pulse rate of 120.

② Regular abdominal breathing.

③ Flaccidity of the lower extremities.

④ Crying in response to being physically stimulated.

Flaccidity of the lower extremities would receive a 0 rating on the APGAR scoring of muscle tone. Thus, the highest possible score Baby Boy Wilson could receive would be an 8 out of a possible 10 points. Correct answer ③.

52. Three of the following drugs may be administered to Ms. Wilson while she is in the delivery room. Which one would **NOT** be given to her since she is planning to breast feed her infant?

① Oxytocin injection (Pitocin).

② Ergonovine maleate (Ergotrate).

③ Methylergonovine (Methergine) maleate.

④ Testosterone enanthate and estradiol valerate (Deladumone).

Deladumone is a preparation which is administered to postpartum mothers to suppress lactation. Since Ms. Wilson is planning to breast feed it is not advisable for her to receive this medication. Correct answer ④.

53. Ms. Wilson expresses concern about her ability to supply the baby with enough milk because of his large size. Which of these ideas should most certainly be included in the nurse's response?

① Supplemental feedings can be added for babies who weigh more than 9 pounds.

② Eight to ten glasses of fluid per day, half of which should be milk, will insure an adequate milk supply.

③ Smoking should be avoided since it interferes with blood circulation in the mammary glands, thus reducing milk production.

④ The more the baby sucks, the more milk the breasts will produce to meet the baby's needs.

Breast feeding is based on supply and demand. Therefore, the more the baby sucks, the more milk is produced. The sucking and emptying of the breast stimulates release of hormones which signal milk production. Correct answer ④.

54. Ms. Wilson asks the nurse how effective oral contraceptive drugs are in preventing pregnancy. Which of these replies would be accurate?

① "They are quite effective in women whose menstrual cycle is regular."

② "They vary in effectiveness according to the woman's age."

③ "They are very effective when taken exactly as prescribed."

④ "They are highly effective only if used in conjunction with a birth control device such as a diaphragm."

Oral contraceptives are approximately 99% effective when taken as directed. The best answer is ③. The factors mentioned in the other answers do not influence the effectiveness of oral contraceptives. Correct answer ③.

Ms. Mary Varnick is a 25-year-old multigravida who is 8 months pregnant. She comes to the hospital and is admitted to the labor room with bright red vaginal bleeding. The physician suspects that Ms. Varnick may have placenta previa or abruptio placentae.

---

55. During the admission process, three of the following measures would be appropriate for Ms. Varnick. Which one would be **contraindicated** for her?

① Giving an enema.

② Obtaining a urine specimen.

③ Checking for uterine contractions.

④ Shaving the perineal area.

Until an assessment of maternal status can be made, it would be best to avoid rectal or vaginal procedures. These manipulations could stimulate further bleeding and preterm labor. Correct answer ①.

56. When Ms. Varnick is admitted, which of the following information should be obtained **first**?

① Her temperature and respiratory rate.

② Her blood pressure and pulse rate.

③ Her height and weight.

④ The date of her last menstrual period and the dates of her previous pregnancies.

Since Ms. Varnick has bright red vaginal bleeding the nurse needs to assess her for symptoms of hemorrhage. By taking her blood pressure and pulse rate first, a baseline can be established and these signs can be evaluated. In the presence of hemorrhage, hypotension occurs and the pulse becomes weak, rapid and thready. Correct answer ②.

GO ON TO THE NEXT PAGE.

57. The nurse carefully records the symptoms Ms. Varnick describes because this information will help the physician confirm a diagnosis. Ms. Varnick is more likely to have abruptio placentae than placenta previa if she complains of

① thirst.

② projectile vomiting.

③ abdominal pain.

④ small cysts in the vaginal discharge.

Vaginal bleeding accompanied by abdominal pain is the primary external sign of abruptio placenta. Correct answer ③.

It is determined that Ms. Varnick has placenta previa, and a cesarean section is performed under spinal anesthesia. A 4-lb. (1,814-gm.) girl is delivered and is transferred to the premature nursery, where she is placed in an incubator. Ms. Varnick is transferred from the recovery room to the postpartum unit with an intravenous infusion in her left arm and an indwelling urinary catheter attached to gravity drainage.

---

58. Identification tags were placed on both Baby Girl Varnick and her mother before they left the delivery room. The chief reason this was done at that time is that

① it is the recommended hospital policy.

② it is the most convenient time.

③ the procedure can be done under aseptic conditions.

④ the baby and her mother had not yet been separated.

Immediate application of identification tags lessens the possibility of error in the identification process. Since there is but one mother and one baby in the delivery room the margin for error is reduced. Correct answer ④.

59. Ms. Varnick is to be kept flat in bed for about 8 hours postoperatively. The purpose of this measure is to prevent

① headache.

② hemorrhage.

③ hypertension.

④ pulmonary embolus.

Headache is sometimes a complication after spinal anesthesia. Headache occurs when there is decreased intracranial pressure which may be brought on by standing in an upright position. Correct answer ①.

60. An hour after Ms. Varnick is transferred to the postpartum unit, the nurse notes that her blood pressure reading has changed from 120/80 to 96/70 and that her abdominal dressings are dry.

Which of these actions should the nurse take first?

① Massage Ms. Varnick's uterine fundus.

② Elevate the foot of Ms. Varnick's bed.

③ Check Ms. Varnick's perineal pad.

④ Change Ms. Varnick's position.

The nurse has recognized the symptoms of hermorrage and wisely checked the abdominal dressings. The nurse needs to be aware that the client may be hemorrhaging via the vagina and should also check the perineal pad and assess the amount of lochia. Correct answer ③.

61. Ms. Varnick's indwelling urinary catheter is removed at 10 a.m. on the day after delivery. The time and amount of each of Ms. Varnick's first three voidings after the catheter is removed are as follows: 5 p.m., 350 ml.; 11 p.m., 280 ml.; and 6 a.m., 370 ml.

Which of these understandings should the nurse have about Ms. Varnick's urinary pattern?

① The amounts voided and the intervals between voidings are within normal limits.

② The amounts voided are normal, but the intervals between voidings are above normal.

③ The amounts voided are above normal, but the intervals between voidings are normal.

④ The amounts voided and the intervals between voidings are below normal.

Voiding every four to six hours in amounts over 200-250 ml. is considered within the normal range for the postpartum client. Small, frequent voidings could be symptoms of retention and would be cause for concern. Correct answer ①.

62. It is important for the mother of a premature infant to have early contact with her baby because this practice

① reduces the mother's dependency needs.

② stimulates the physical growth rate of the baby.

③ enhances the mother-infant relationship.

④ decreases the likelihood that postpartum blues might occur.

Mother-infant relationships are enhanced if the mother is given the opportunity to touch and hold her infant. Separation increases the mother's anxiety and prevents the mutual interaction which promotes bonding. Correct answer ③.

63. Which of these statements is correct about breast engorgement and afterpains in Ms. Varnick in comparison with multiparas who have delivered vaginally?

① She is likely to have breast engorgement and afterpains similar to those of women who delivered vaginally.

② She is likely to have afterpains similar to those of women who delivered vaginally, but breast engorgement will be absent.

③ Her breast engorgement will be similar to that of women who delivered vaginally, but afterpains will be absent.

④ Her breast engorgement and her afterpains will be different from those of women who delivered vaginally.

Postpartal changes which affect the breast and uterus are experienced equally by mothers regardless of the method of delivery. Cesarean section clients differ from vaginal delivery clients in that they may have less lochia. Correct answer ①.

64. On Ms. Varnick's sixth postpartum day, her lochia is bright red and moderate in amount. Which of these actions should the nurse take first?

① Encourage Ms. Varnick to increase her ambulation in order to aid involution.

② Have Ms. Varnick lie on her abdomen for about an hour in order to apply pressure to the uterus.

③ Chart the observation.

④ Report the observation to the nurse in charge.

Bright red moderate lochia on the sixth day postpartum is a deviation from normal. Lochia should be pink, serous, and blood tinged from day 4 until day 7 to 10. The correct answer is to report this finding to the charge nurse for further assessment. Correct answer ④.

The next section of the test consists of individual questions relating to maternity nursing.

---

65. The nurse should be alert to symptoms characteristic of severe preeclampsia, which include

① ringing in the ears and rapid pulse.

② elevated temperature and excitability.

③ vomiting and excessive urination.

④ persistent headache and blurred vision.

Preeclampsia is caused by hypertension. The nurse recognizes persistent headaches and blurred vision as signs of elevated blood pressure. Correct answer ④.

66. In the care of a newborn with hydrocephalus, which of these measures is especially important?

① Keeping the baby dry.

② Changing the baby's position at regular intervals.

③ Feeding the baby small amounts of formula frequently.

④ Placing the baby so that his head is lower than the rest of his body.

It is important to change the baby's position at regular intervals to prevent the development of pressure sores on the baby's head. If his head is very enlarged, the baby may not be able to turn it independently. Correct answer ②.

67. A newborn who has a cleft palate is to be bottle fed. Which of these measures would it be most important to take when feeding this infant?

① Applying elbow restraints to the infant prior to each feeding.

② Holding the infant in an upright position during feedings.

③ Giving the infant a small amount of sterile water after each feeding.

④ Feeding the infant small amounts frequently.

Holding the infant in an upright position during feeding facilitates swallowing, burping and retention of formula. It also prevents aspiration or vomiting. Correct answer ②.

The next section of the test consists of questions relating to the care of children.

Steve Holmes, 8 years old, has sickle cell anemia. He is admitted to the hospital in sickle cell crisis.

---

68. As the nurse is transporting Steve from the emergency room to the pediatric unit, he asks why he gets sick. The nurse shares Steve's question with the staff of the pediatric unit.

The explanation Steve is given should be based on the information that sickle cell anemia is caused by

① genetic factors.

② antigen-antibody reactions.

③ nutritional deficiencies.

④ metabolic disorders.

Communication with clients and with other staff members is vital. All involved with sickle cell anemia must understand that it is caused by a genetically inherited deficit in the formation of hemaglobin. If both parents carry this recessive trait, the child will show symptoms as early as 2 months of age. Correct answer ①.

GO ON TO THE NEXT PAGE.

69. Steve is complaining of pain in his legs and abdomen. Steve's mother is concerned and asks the nurse what causes the pain. The nurse's response is based on the understanding that such pain is the result of

① bleeding into the cellular spaces.

② clumping of erythrocytes.

③ a generalized infectious process.

④ a shift of intestinal fluid.

Steve's pain results from clumping of erythrocytes. This condition results in occlusion of capillaries which decreases oxygen to the cells. The mother has a right to know about her child's disease and treatment. The nurse can best explain Steve's complaints in terms his mother will understand. Correct answer ②.

70. Steve is very quiet and lies facing the wall much of the time. Which of these measures by the nurse would be best?

① Spending time with Steve other than when giving him physical care.

② Providing Steve with an opportunity to talk with an older child who also has sickle cell anemia.

③ Assuring Steve at frequent intervals that he is improving.

④ Reminding Steve that being upset might make his condition worse.

Steve, at age 8, may be scared and uncertain of what will happen during his hospitalization. Spending time with him when physical care is not being given will show Steve that the nurse's interest is not only in his disease and will give the opportunity to discuss his fears and concerns. Correct answer ①.

71. Ms. Holmes says to the nurse, "I hope Steve will stop having these crises." The nurse's response should be based on which of these understandings?

① Sickle cell anemia can be controlled if the disease is diagnosed at birth.

② Sickle cell anemia is a chronic disease characterized by periods of crisis throughout life.

③ If the child with sickle cell anemia is in remission for two years, the disease is considered arrested.

④ If the child with sickle cell anemia reaches puberty, the crises will no longer occur.

At this time there is no cure for sickle cell anemia and the course of the disease varies for each client. It is a chronic disease with crises occurring throughout the client's lifetime at different intervals. It is not considered to be arrested regardless of the time between crises or the age of the client. Correct answer ②.

72. Which of these understandings about children of Steve's age (8 years) should the nurse keep in mind when planning their play activities?

① They need to have highly structured activities.

② They prefer being with children of the opposite sex.

③ They like to be involved with a group of children their own age.

④ They usually include an imaginary playmate in their activities.

Children, at age 8, show a definite preference for group play with children their own age of both sexes. They can structure their own activities and have outgrown the imaginary playmate stage. Correct answer ③.

Steve's condition improves, and plans are made with Mr. and Ms. Holmes for his discharge.

73. Ms. Holmes says to the nurse, "We're planning to go camping at a lake for the entire summer. It's about four hundred miles from here." Because Steve has sickle cell anemia, which of these suggestions would it be appropriate for the nurse to make to Ms. Holmes?

① "Be sure that Steve is not exposed to the sun."

② "Plan to drive for only short periods at a time so that Steve will have a chance to exercise his legs."

③ "Limit Steve's fluids while traveling to help prevent him from being carsick."

④ "Ask your physician about the medical facilities that are available where you are going."

Whenever a change of location is anticipated, the client and the client's family need to know the type and location of medical care facilities available should a sickle cell crisis occur. Correct answer ④.

Harry Shapiro, 12 years old, is brought to the emergency room by his parents. A diagnosis of acute appendicitis is made and Harry is scheduled for surgery.

An appendectomy is performed. Because the appendix had ruptured, a drain is inserted in the incision. Harry is brought to the pediatric unit with an intravenous infusion running. He has a nasogastric tube connected to intermittent suction.

74. A nasogastric tube may be inserted for three of the following purposes. Which one is the **exception**?

① To relieve distention.

② To re-establish normal peristalsis.

③ To facilitate drainage from the stomach.

④ To allow for the measurement of stomach contents.

Following bowel surgery it is advisable to keep the bowel deflated and allow it time to heal. The nasogastric tube is used for this purpose. It prevents establishment of normal peristalsis since the stimulus for peristaltic movement is the distention of the bowel. Correct answer ②.

GO ON TO THE NEXT PAGE.

75. An antibiotic has been added to Harry's intravenous fluids to treat the existing peritonitis. The nurse understands that she must assess Harry for untoward effects of the drug. Which of the following is a common symptom of an antibiotic hypersensitivity?

① Anorexia.

② Urticaria.

③ Constipation.

④ Hypertension.

A rash or urticaria is a common symptom of an antibiotic drug reaction. Other symptoms are hypotension, vomiting, diarrhea, respiratory distress and, most seriously, anaphylaxis. Correct answer ②.

76. In the early postoperative period, which of these understandings about administering medication for pain to children such as Harry is accurate?

① Analgesia is usually necessary and is safe if the dosage is calculated for the individual child.

② Potential drug addiction should be a major concern in the care of an acutely ill child.

③ Since children are active earlier in the postoperative period than adults, they will need little or no analgesia.

④ Children have a higher tolerance for pain than do adults and therefore need smaller doses of drugs.

Children, as well as adults, may require analgesia following surgery. However, when children are medicated the dosage is smaller and needs to be calculated according to the child's individual body weight. Correct answer ①.

77. Which of these behaviors is characteristic of most normal 12-year-olds?

① Rejection of new routines.

② Shyness when meeting new people.

③ Anxiety caused by separation from parents.

④ Embarrassment associated with elimination.

A 12-year-old is entering puberty and may be self-conscious about secondary sexual characteristics which are developing. Therefore, the nurse needs to be careful to insure privacy for a 12-year-old during elimination. Correct answer ④.

Linda Malone, a 3-month-old infant with two siblings, is brought by her mother to the clinic for routine health care. Linda has some localized scaling and red areas on her cheeks, neck, and elbows, which are diagnosed as eczema.

78. Which of these suggestions regarding Linda's care is it most important for the nurse to give Ms. Malone?

① Bathe Linda daily with a mild soap.

② Keep Linda's nails cut short.

③ Use only long-sleeved clothing for Linda.

④ Have the other children in the family avoid contact with Linda.

Since itching may be intense in the child with eczema, Linda will try to scratch herself. Keeping her fingernails cut short will lessen the chance of secondary infection developing. Correct answer ②.

79. Which of these behaviors should the nurse expect to observe in a normal 3-month-old infant?

① Holding the bottle during a feeding.

② Smiling in response to being talked to.

③ Turning from the back to the abdomen.

④ Crying when a stranger approaches.

A normal 3-month-old will respond with a smile when spoken to. Correct answer ②.

Linda's eczema remains under control until she is 6 months of age. She is then admitted to the hospital because of a severe flare-up of the eczema on her arms and trunk.

---

80. Linda is wearing elbow restraints. At which of these times would it be most appropriate to remove her restraints?

① When she is being held.

② When she is sleeping.

③ When she is being wheeled in a carriage around the unit.

④ When the nurse is in her room.

Linda's elbow restraints can be removed when she is being held. When an adult is holding her, she is restrained naturally. She can move freely and have the advantage of being touched, while still being prevented from scratching the areas of eczema. Correct answer ①.

81. Linda is receiving an antihistamine. The purpose of this medication is to

① promote healing of the lesions.

② reduce itching of the lesions.

③ limit the spread of the lesions.

④ prevent infection of the lesions.

Eczema is considered to be essentially an allergic response and one of the symptoms is itching that may be reduced with antihistamines. Correct answer ②.

GO ON TO THE NEXT PAGE.

Linda is discharged. When she is 1 year old, she is readmitted to the hospital with another flare-up of the eczema.

82. Which of these recent changes in Linda's life is most likely related to the increased severity of her eczema?

① A new foam-rubber mattress was placed in her crib.

② Eggs were included in her diet for the first time.

③ Her parents had their home air-conditioned.

④ She has a new cotton blanket on her bed.

The most common causes of allergies are foods that are protein in nature. Eggs are classified as a common food that may cause an allergic reaction. Correct answer ②.

83. The nurse is asked to record Linda's developmental abilities. Linda has all the following abilities. Which one was probably acquired most recently?

① Sitting for extended periods without support.

② Transferring a toy from one hand to the other.

③ Sitting down from a standing position without help.

④ Rolling over completely.

Motor development occurs in an orderly progression from the simple to the complex as the nervous system matures. Sitting down from a standing position is the most complex of the activities and would, therefore, be the one most recently acquired. Correct answer ③.

Claire Menard, 4 months old, is admitted to the hospital with severe diarrhea and dehydration. Isolation precautions are instituted. She is to receive nothing by mouth. Ms. Menard plans to spend each afternoon with Claire.

84. For which of these purposes is it **most** important to weigh Claire when she is admitted to the unit?

① To assess the seriousness of her condition.

② To determine the presence of edema.

③ To compare her weight with the normal range for her age.

④ To calculate her fluid requirements.

Weighing Claire will provide a useful assessment of water loss and a basis for calculating her fluid requirements. Correct answer ④.

85. For which of these purposes is Claire to receive nothing by mouth?

① To reduce the spread of disease-producing organisms.
② To provide for a more accurate measurement of stool volume.
③ To prevent aspiration.
④ To decrease activity in the gastrointestinal tract.

Ingestion of food stimulates gastrointestinal activity and increases diarrhea. Initial treatment requires letting bowel rest. Correct answer ④.

Claire is receiving intravenous fluids.

86. Claire's intravenous equipment is to be adjusted so that she receives 18 microdrops per minute. The nurse notices that only 2 microdrops are being delivered per minute.

Before reporting this observation to the nurse in charge, which of these actions should the nurse take?

① Milk the intravenous tubing.
② Check the site of the intravenous infusion.
③ Open the clamp on the intravenous tubing completely.
④ Raise the intravenous bottle.

The nurse should check the site of the intravenous infusion for infiltration. If the site is swollen and painful, infiltration is indicated. Correct answer ②.

87. The nurse should be aware that if Claire's intravenous infusion were to run too fast, which of these complications would be most likely to occur?

① Severe diarrhea.
② Thrombus formation.
③ Renal failure.
④ Circulatory overload.

Circulatory overload occurs if the intravenous infusion delivers too much fluid too fast. Correct answer ④.

88. Claire's mother, Ms. Menard, asks the nurse what she could do to be helpful to Claire. Which of these suggestions should the nurse give to Ms. Menard?

① "Write down the number of stools Claire has."
② "Keep track of the fluid in Claire's I.V. bottle."
③ "Caress Claire frequently when she is awake."
④ "Remind me when it is time to change Claire's position."

Caressing Claire frequently when she is awake will reinforce mother-child bonding and intimacy and will be therapeutic for both. Correct answer ③.

GO ON TO THE NEXT PAGE.

Claire's condition improves and she is started on oral feedings.

89. The nurse is to feed Claire for the first time. Which of these measures should be taken in relation to the feeding situation?

① Giving Claire a small amount of the feeding at a time.

② Holding Claire in an upright position during the feeding.

③ Bubbling Claire each time she has taken a half ounce of the feeding.

④ Positioning Claire with her head slightly lower than her chest after feeding her.

Claire should receive a small amount of feeding at a time initially to check tolerance. As Claire's condition improves the amount of feeding can be increased. Correct answer ①.

90. Claire is to be weighed daily. At which of these times would it be best to weigh her?

① Prior to her first morning feeding.

② After she has been bathed.

③ After her first bowel movement of the day.

④ Whenever her mother is available to assist with the procedure.

Claire should be weighed prior to her first feeding daily. Measurement at this time will provide accurate information about Claire's condition and progress. Correct answer ①.

Bobby Tate, 20 months old, is to be admitted to the hospital for surgical repair of an inguinal hernia.

91. The nurse is asked to assist with Bobby's admission by recording his symptoms. These will include which common symptom of an inguinal hernia?

① Protrusion of the umbilicus.

② Visible peristalsis.

③ A mass in the groin.

④ Abdominal distention.

If the tube formed by a sac of peritoneum does not atrophy after the descent of the testis in utero, the intestine may descend into that sac and produce an inguinal hernia. The hernia is a visible mass in the groin. Correct answer ③.

92. Bobby arrives at the hospital clutching a rather soiled, ragged baby blanket. When his mother attempts to remove the blanket to take it home, Bobby cries and holds on to it.

Which of these comments by the nurse would indicate the best understanding of Bobby's needs?

① "It looks as if that's Bobby's favorite blanket. It's all right for him to keep it with him."

② "Let's wait until Bobby is involved in an activity, and then I'll take the blanket and give it to you next time you come."

③ "I'll get Bobby another blanket. Then he won't mind giving up this one."

④ "Tell Bobby that you only want to take the blanket to wash it and that you'll bring it back next time you come."

At 20 months, children are frequently attached to objects. The object becomes extremely important, particularly if the child is frightened. The comment that best indicates the nurse's understanding of such an attachment is, "It looks as if that's Bobby's favorite blanket. It is all right for him to keep it with him." Correct answer ①.

93. Bobby is to have a venipuncture to obtain a blood specimen. When the physician is ready to take Bobby's blood, which of these approaches by the nurse would be best?

① Tell Bobby which arm to extend to the physician.

② Hold Bobby's arm in position for the physician.

③ Show Bobby how to squeeze his fist tight while the needle is being inserted.

④ Have Bobby cover his eyes with one hand while the specimen is being withdrawn.

A child of 20 months cannot be expected to remain still during a painful procedure. To insure a quick, successful venipuncture, it is important that the nurse hold Bobby's arm firmly in position. Correct answer ②.

94. Ms. Tate tells the nurse that she has to leave because she has a 6-month-old baby at home. Ms. Tate says, "Bobby has never been away from home without me and I think he's going to be very upset."

Which of these responses by the nurse would be best?

① "Maybe if you promise to bring him his favorite toy when you return, he won't cry so much."

② "If we hear Bobby crying, we will send someone in to care for him."

③ "I'll stay here with Bobby and try to comfort him."

④ "Most children only cry for a little while after their mothers leave."

It is normal for Bobby to cry when his mother leaves. Bobby's mother needs to be reassured that someone will be with her child to comfort him. "I'll stay here with Bobby and try to comfort him," is the best response. Correct answer ③.

Bobby is scheduled for surgery and is to have nothing by mouth.

95. While Bobby can have nothing by mouth, he is unhappy and cries for something to drink. Which of these measures would it be appropriate to include in his care?

① Taking Bobby for a walk.

② Giving Bobby chips of ice to suck.

③ Having Bobby use a pleasant-flavored mouthwash.

④ Explaining to Bobby why he cannot have fluids.

Bobby will be unhappy and thirsty when he cannot drink. While mouthwash and an explanation might work well for an adult or older child, Bobby will not understand and he may swallow the mouthwash. Ice cannot be given to anyone who is to have nothing by mouth. Taking Bobby for a walk is the most appropriate intervention because distraction is an effective technique for dealing with a 20-month-old. Correct answer ①.

Bobby has surgery. He is to be discharged the next day.

96. Ms. Tate tells the nurse that Bobby does not drink enough milk. Which of these foods is the best substitute for milk?

① Citrus fruit juices.

② Cream.

③ Cheese.

④ Root vegetables.

Cheese is a good milk substitute. It contains large amounts of calcium and is not as high in calories as cream. Citrus juices and root vegetables do not offer the protein of milk. Correct answer ③.

Anna Garcia, 2 years old, is admitted to the hospital with a diagnosis of laryngotracheobronchitis. She is placed in a croup tent with oxygen.

97. Ms. Garcia asks why her daughter has been placed in the croup tent. The nurse explains that Anna will be more comfortable because the tent will relieve which of the following symptoms of laryngotracheobronchitis?

① Wheezing.

② Dyspnea.

③ Swelling of the neck.

④ Protusion of the tongue.

Laryngotracheobronchitis is the result of a sudden change in condition of young children who have a mild upper respiratory infection. The child has severe dyspnea caused by edema of the mucous membrane and copious, thick mucus. Correct answer ②.

98. The nurse is unable to count Anna's respirations accurately because she is restless and crying. Which of these actions by the nurse would be best?

① Ask another staff member to count Anna's respirations.

② Record an approximate respiratory rate.

③ Postpone taking Anna's respirations until she becomes quiet.

④ Average her respirations per minute after taking them for 3 minutes.

Every effort should be made to avoid further aggravation of Anna's respiratory distress. The nurse should postpone taking respirations until the child becomes quiet. Correct answer ③.

99. The evening after Anna's admission, Ms. Garcia arrives to visit Anna. Ms. Garcia says to the nurse, "I just put my hand in the tent. Anna's clothing is damp."

In addition to changing Anna's clothing, which of these actions should the nurse take in response to Ms. Garcia's comment?

① Report Ms. Garcia's observation to the nurse in charge.

② Encourage Anna to drink fluids to replace those she is losing.

③ Take Anna's temperature to compare it with her previous temperature.

④ Explain the function of the humidity to Ms. Garcia.

The nurse should explain to Ms. Garcia that the function of the croup tent is to generate high humidity to aid in thinning respiratory secretions. The dampness of Anna's clothing is due to condensation and is nothing to be alarmed about. Correct answer ④.

100. Licensed practical nurses are responsible for monitoring clients receiving oxygen therapy. To meet this responsibility, the nurse should know that the outcome of oxygen therapy is to

① increase the respiratory and pulse rates.

② increase the respiratory rate and reduce the pulse rate.

③ reduce the respiratory rate and increase the pulse rate.

④ reduce the respiratory and pulse rates.

Increased respirations and pulse are symptoms of hypoxemia. Oxygen relieves these symptoms. Correct answer ④.

GO ON TO THE NEXT PAGE.

Anna's condition improves, and she is to be removed from the croup tent for short periods during the day.

101. Before returning Anna to the croup tent, the nurse should take which of these actions?

① Close the tent and turn on the oxygen flow meter.

② Wipe the inside of the canopy with a disinfectant solution.

③ Give Anna fluids to drink.

④ Assist Anna in doing deep-breathing exercises.

One of the safety rules of oxygen administration is to "flush" enclosed units with oxygen before placing the client inside them. Correct answer ①.

Anna's condition has improved. She is ambulatory and is to be discharged soon.

102. Anna is in the playroom. Which of these behaviors is typical of a 2-year-old child?

① Playing a simple board game with another child of the same age.

② Sitting quietly with a group of children while listening to a story.

③ Coloring within the lines of drawings in a coloring book, using jumbo-size crayons.

④ Engaging in activities near other children but not with them.

The 2-year-old child engages in parallel play, that is, playing alongside but not actually with other children. Correct answer ④.

103. Ms. Garcia tells the nurse that for the past month Anna has not been eating as much as usual and that she is eating less than her 1-year-old brother. The most likely reason for this change in Anna's appetite is

① dislike of the food she is being given.

② a decrease in her growth rate.

③ jealousy of her brother.

④ a reluctance to feed herself.

The average weight gain in the second year of life is approximately 5 lbs., whereas at the end of the first year the birth weight normally triples. Correct answer ②.

104. When Anna is ready for discharge, Ms. Garcia asks the nurse what she should do if Anna begins to develop symptoms of croup again. Which of these questions would it be best to ask Ms. Garcia **initially**?

① "Has anyone ever showed you how to do postural drainage with Anna?"

② "How far from your home is the nearest emergency room?"

③ "Does rocking Anna or singing to her help to relax her?"

④ "Does your bathroom steam up easily when you run the hot water?"

If the bathroom steams up easily, the mother can put the child in the room and run the hot water. The humidity will reduce respiratory spasms. Since some children who develop croup tend to have future episodes, the mother should know what to do when the child has symptoms at home. Correct answer ④.

The next section of the test consists of individual questions relating to the care of children.

---

105. In order to accomplish toilet training with a minimum of conflict for the child and the parent, which of these methods by the parent would be best?

① Put the child on the toilet after breakfast and have him stay there until his bowels move.

② Put the child on the toilet and promise him candy when his bowels move.

③ Disapprove of the child each time he soils himself.

④ Start toileting the child when he begins fussing about soiling his diapers.

Toilet training should begin when a child develops awareness of his discomfort after incontinent bowel and bladder emptying and wants to do something about it. Correct answer ④.

106. Rose, 2 years old, is to receive an antibiotic orally in liquid form. Before pouring the medication, it is essential for the nurse to

① wipe the lip of the container with a sterile cotton ball.

② hold the bottle under warm running water for a few seconds.

③ find out if Rose has ever taken a liquid medication.

④ shake the bottle well if there is a precipitate.

In order for Rose to get the correct amount of prescribed antibiotic, the nurse must shake the bottle well to make sure that there is no precipitate. Correct answer ④.

107. An 11-year-old boy who is in a spica cast often eats too much and then complains of discomfort. Which of these measures is likely to be most helpful to him concerning this problem?

① Giving him smaller but more frequent meals.

② Continuing to give him three meals a day, but giving him smaller portions.

③ Restricting his fluid intake.

④ Encouraging him to eat slowly and to alternate liquids with solids.

Small, frequent feedings will prevent discomfort. The nurse should instruct the boy about smaller portions to insure his understanding and cooperation. Correct answer ①.

The last section of the test consists of general individual questions.

---

108. A worker who is putting up a metal partition on the surgical unit goes to a nurse on the unit and says that he just got a metal fragment in his eye. Which of these actions by the nurse would demonstrate the best judgment?

① Find out if the man has pain in the unaffected eye.

② Irrigate the man's affected eye with sterile water.

③ Examine the man's affected eye.

④ Send the man to the emergency room.

Sending the man to the emergency room is the most appropriate action. Early detection and treatment of an eye injury may prevent permanent damage and disability. Correct answer ④.

109. Which of these practices is generally **unacceptable** in recording on a client's chart?

① Using abbreviations.

② Using incomplete sentences or phrases.

③ Making erasures.

④ Recording subjective symptoms.

Making erasures is unacceptable. Hospital policy and procedure regarding documentation are good guidelines for acceptable and unacceptable notations on a client's chart. Correct answer ③.

110. A client is to receive regular insulin, 40 units of U-100 insulin. Only protamine zinc insulin (PZI) U-100 is available on the unit. The nurse gives the patient 40 units of PZI.

Which of these evaluations of the nurse's action is most justifiable?

① The action was appropriate because these preparations of insulin are the same strength.

② The action was appropriate because these preparations of insulin have similar properties.

③ The action was inappropriate because the replacement of one preparation of insulin with another is not a function of nursing.

④ The action was inappropriate because regular insulin is less concentrated and a smaller dose of PZI is required.

Making decisions about insulin dosage and preparation are the physician's responsibility. In this case the nurse's action was inappropriate. Correct answer ③.

111. One day the nurse notices that a male worker who ordinarily does not have access to the medicine cabinet is unlocking the cabinet and looking through the contents on the shelves.

Which of these actions by the nurse would be best?

① Tell the worker that he is not authorized to open the cabinet without supervision.

② Demand the keys from the worker and lock the cabinet.

③ Report the incident to the nurse in charge immediately.

④ Ask the worker where he obtained the keys to the cabinet.

Immediately reporting the incident to the nurse in charge is the best action. The charge nurse is responsible for the management of the ward and can best handle the problem. Correct answer ③.

112. The nurse has a responsibility to collect and accurately record information on clients' charts. This information could ethically be shared in all but one of the following situations. In which one would it be **unethical**?

① At a conference with the unit supervisor.

② At a conference sponsored by a practical nurse association.

③ At a team conference with members of allied health groups.

④ At a clinical conference for staff members.

Sharing information with others involved in a client's care is necessary for planning and implementing adequate care, but the Practical Nurses' Code of Ethics and the Patient's Bill of Rights both insure confidentiality. A conference sponsored by a practical nurse association is a public forum and those attending should not be privy to specific information about a named client. Correct answer ②.

113. An elderly client who is in the hospital convalescing from surgery asks for the nurse's help in writing a will. Which of these actions would it be best for the nurse to take?

① Contact a lawyer for the patient.

② Inform the client's family of the patient's desire.

③ Tell the client that a will written in the hospital is not valid.

④ Report the request to the nurse in charge.

Reporting the request to the charge nurse is the most appropriate action. The charge nurse is responsible for handling the situation. Correct answer ④.

This is the end of the test.

Before handing in your answer sheet, make certain that you have

1. answered all the questions to which you think you know the correct answer.
2. erased all stray or accidental marks in your test booklet.
3. filled in all the information requested.

Appendix

Administration of Examination Committee Testing Dates

NCLEX for *Registered Nurse* Licensure —

1985:	February 5– 6 and July 16–17
1986:	February 4– 5 and July 15–16
1987:	February 3– 4 and July 14–15
1988:	February 2– 3 and July 12–13
1989:	February 14–15 and July 11–12
1990:	February 6– 7 and July 10–11
1991:	February 5– 6 and July 9–10
1992:	February 5– 6 and July 8– 9
1993:	February 3– 4 and July 7– 8
1994:	February 2– 3 and July 13–14

NCLEX for *Practical Nurse* Licensure —

1985:	April 16 and October 15
1986:	April 15 and October 21
1987:	April 7 and October 20
1988:	April 19 and October 18
1989:	April 18 and October 17
1990:	April 17 and October 16
1991:	April 16 and October 15
1992:	April 15 and October 21
1993:	April 14 and October 13
1994:	April 13 and October 12

Constructing the National Council Examinations for Licensure

- EC revises/recommends acceptance of Test Plans

- DA adopts new Test Plan

- PTS reviews items in pool to determine needs of Test Plan specifications and refers needs to EC

- EC refers needs for IW to NCSBN Board of Directors

- BD selects IW from nominees submitted by Member Boards of Nursing representing approximately 12–14 jurisdictions for RN and 12–14 jurisdictions for PN per year

  > **Selection** — Based on qualifications, regional distribution, type of program and clinical practice. Boards submit nominees on a regularly scheduled basis and may participate more frequently if preferred.

- EC gives confidential directions to IW

- IW participate in training and item writing workshop. IW with PTS validate, edit, and classify items according to Test Plan

- PTS edits and validates items for agreement with examination specifications, psychometric properties, documentation, ethnic and sexual bias, accuracy in classification and grammar

- BD selects PCE from nominees submitted by Member Boards of Nursing representing approximately 12–14 jurisdictions for RN and 12–14 jurisdictions for PN

  > **Selection** — Based on qualifications, regional distribution, and clinical practice. Boards submit nominees on a regularly scheduled basis and may participate more frequently if preferred.

- PTS conducts meeting of each PCE including a representative of EC

- PCE reviews appropriateness of each new item and pool items requiring updating review. Review includes documentation of content accuracy, currency, job-relatedness, appropriateness for entry-level, verification of correct answer for each item, and disposition

- PTS assembles experimental items for try-out as directed by PCE

- MB files a request to review experimental items. Review experimental items for appropriateness for entry-level practice and consistency with laws regulating nursing practice in the jurisdictions

- PTS collates responses of Member Boards and conducts statistical analysis of "try-out" items

- PCE reviews responses from Member Boards and statistical analysis of "try-out" items and decides outcome of items

- EC writes confidential directions for PTS in assembling the examination which includes "real" and "try-out" items

- PTS assembles examination for administration including both "real" and "try-out" items

- EC reviews examination for administration in series and form approved for use

KEY

EC — Examination Committee of the National Council of State Boards of Nursing, Inc. Members represent the areas of the National Council. One additional registered nurse employee of a separate board of practical nursing participants in activities related to the examination for practical nurse licensure.

PTS — Professional Test Service under contract with the National Council.

BD — Board of Directors of the National Council of State Boards of Nursing, Inc. Members represent the areas of the National Council and are elected by the National Council members.

Series and Form — Series refers to the NCLEX for Registered Nurse Licensure, and Form refers to the NCLEX for Practical Nurse Licensure.

PCE — Panel of Content Experts. Members are nominated by Member Boards annually. These content experts will review items to assure that understandings basic to minimum safe and effective practice are being evaluated for entry level practical nurses.

DA — Delegate Assembly of NCSBN. Consists of representatives from each jurisdiction who govern the National Council.

IW — Item Writers. Individuals who are nominated by Member Boards and appointed by NCSBN Board of Directors.

NCSBN — National Council of State Boards of Nursing, Inc.

MB — Member Boards. Boards of Nursing in those jurisdictions which are members of the National Council of State Boards of Nursing, Inc.

State and Territorial Boards of Nursing and Practical Nursing

ALABAMA
Executive Officer
Alabama Board of Nursing
Suite 203, 500 Eastern Blvd.
Montgomery, Alabama 36117
Tel: (205) 261-4060

ALASKA
Executive Officer
Alaska Board of Nursing
Dept. of Commerce & Economic
  Development
Div. of Occupational Licensing
The Frontier Bldg.
3601 C Street, Suite 722
Anchorage, Alaska 99502-0333
Tel: (907) 561-2878

For Licensing Information
Licensing Director
Board of Nursing
Pouch "D"
Juneau, Alaska 99811

AMERICAN SAMOA
Executive Secretary
American Samoa Health Service
  Regulatory Board
Pago Pago, American Samoa 96799
Tel: (684) 633-1222 ext. 206

ARIZONA
Executive Secretary
Arizona State Board of Nursing
State Occupational Licensing Bldg.
5050 N. 19th Ave., Suite 103
Phoenix, Arizona 85015
Tel: (602) 255-5092

ARKANSAS
Executive Director
Arkansas State Board of Nursing
Westmark Bldg., Suite 308
4120 W. Markham Street
Little Rock, Arkansas 72205
Tel: (501) 371-2751

CALIFORNIA
Executive Officer
State Board of Registered Nursing
1020 N Street, Room 448
Sacramento, California 95814
Tel: (916) 322-3350

Executive Secretary
Board of Vocational Nurse and
  Psychiatric Technical Examiners
1020 N Street
Sacramento, California 95814
Tel: (916) 445-0793

COLORADO
Program Administrator
Colorado Board of Nursing
State Services Bldg., Room 132
1525 Sherman Street
Denver, Colorado 80203
Tel: (303) 839-2871

CONNECTICUT
Executive Secretary
State Board of Examiners for Nursing
150 Washington Street
Hartford, Connecticut 06106
Tel: (203) 566-1032

DELAWARE
Executive Director
Board of Nursing
Margaret O'Neill Building
P.O. Box 1401
Dover, Delaware 19901
Tel: (302) 736-4752

DISTRICT OF COLUMBIA
President
Registered Nurses' Examining Board
614 H Street, N.W.
Washington, D.C. 20001
Tel: (202) 727-7468

President
Practical Nurses' Examining Board
614 H Street, N.W.
Washington, D.C. 20001
Tel: (202) 727-7468

FLORIDA
Executive Director
Board of Nursing
111 Coastline Drive, East
Jacksonville, Florida 32202
Tel: (904) 359-6331

GEORGIA
Executive Director
Board of Nursing
166 Pryor Street, S.W.
Atlanta, Georgia 30303
Tel: (404) 656-3943

Executive Director
State Board of Licensed
 Practical Nurses
166 Pryor Street, S.W.
Atlanta, Georgia 30303
Tel: (404) 656-3921

For Licensing Information
Joint Secretary
State Examining Boards
166 Pryor Street, S.W.
Atlanta, Georgia 30303
Tel: (404) 656-3900

GUAM
Acting Nurse Examiner Administrator
Guam Board of Nurse Examiners
Dept. of Public Health & Social
 Services
P.O. Box 2816
Agana, Guam 95910
Tel: (671) 734-2783

HAWAII
Executive Secretary
Hawaii Board of Nursing
P.O. Box 3469
Honolulu, Hawaii 96801
Tel: (808) 548-7471

IDAHO
Executive Director
Idaho Board of Nursing
Hall of Mirrors
700 West State Street
Boise, Idaho 83720
Tel: (208) 334-3110

ILLINOIS
Nursing Education Coordinator
Dept. of Registration and Education
320 West Washington Street
3rd Floor
Springfield, Illinois 62786
Tel: (217) 782-4386

INDIANA
President
State Board of Nurses' Registration
 and Nursing Education
Health Professions Service Bureau
964 North Pennsylvania Street
Indianapolis, Indiana 46204
Tel: (317) 232-2960

IOWA
Executive Director
Iowa Board of Nursing
Executive Hills East
1223 East Court
Des Moines, Iowa 50319
Tel: (515) 281-3255

KANSAS
Executive Administrator
Kansas Board of Nursing
503 Kansas Avenue, Suite 330
P.O. Box 1098
Topeka, Kansas 66601
Tel: (913) 296-4929

KENTUCKY
Executive Director
Kentucky Board of Nursing
4010 Dupont Circle, Suite 430
Louisville, Kentucky 40207
Tel: (502) 897-5143

LOUISIANA
Executive Director
Board of Nursing
150 Baronne Street, Room 907
New Orleans, Louisiana 70112
Tel: (504) 568-5464

Executive Director
State Board of Practical Nurse Examiners
4201 ½ Canal Street
New Orleans, Louisiana 70119
Tel: (504) 483-4505

MAINE
Executive Director
Board of Nursing
295 Water Street
Augusta, Maine 04330
Tel: (207) 289-2921

MARYLAND
Executive Director
Board of Examiners of Nurses
201 West Preston Street
Baltimore, Maryland 21201
Tel: (301) 383-2084/2085

MASSACHUSETTS
Executive Secretary
Board of Registration in Nursing
Leverett Saltonstall Bldg.
100 Cambridge Street, Room 1509
Boston, Massachusetts 02202
Tel: (617) 727-3060

MICHIGAN
Nursing Consultant
Board of Nursing
Dept. of Licensing & Regulation
Ottawa Towers North
611 West Ottawa
P.O. Box 30018
Lansing, Michigan 48909
Tel: (517) 373-1600

MINNESOTA
Executive Secretary
Board of Nursing
717 Delaware Street, S.E.
Minneapolis, Minnesota 55414
Tel: (612) 623-5493

MISSISSIPPI
Executive Director
Board of Nursing
135 Bounds Street, Suite 101
Jackson, Mississippi 39206
Tel: (601) 354-7349

MISSOURI
Executive Director
Board of Nursing
P.O. Box 656
3423 N. Ten Mile Drive
Jefferson City, Missouri 65102
Tel: (314) 751-2334

MONTANA
Executive Secretary
State Board of Nursing
Dept. of Commerce
Div. of Business & Professional Licensing
1424 9th Avenue
Helena, Montana 59620-0407
Tel: (406) 444-4279

NEBRASKA
Nursing Education Consultant
Board of Nursing
Bureau of Examining Boards
Dept. of Health
State House Station, Box 95065
Lincoln, Nebraska 68509
Tel: (402) 471-2001

NEVADA
Executive Director
Board of Nursing
1135 Terminal Way, Suite 209
Reno, Nevada 89502
Tel: (702) 786-2778

NEW HAMPSHIRE
Executive Director
Board of Nursing Education
    and Nurse Registration
State Dept. of Education
State Office Park South
101 Pleasant Street
Concord, New Hampshire 03301
Tel: (603) 271-2323

NEW JERSEY
Executive Director
Board of Nursing
1100 Raymond Blvd., Room 319
Newark, New Jersey 07102
Tel: (201) 648-2570

NEW MEXICO
Executive Director
Board of Nursing
5301 Central, N.E., Suite 905
Albuquerque, New Mexico 87108
Tel: (505) 841-4620

NEW YORK
Executive Secretary
State Board of Nursing
State Education Dept.
Cultural Education Center
Room 3013
Albany, New York 12230
Tel: (518) 474-3843/3844/3845

For Licensing Information
Supervisor
Div. of Professional Licensing
  Services
State Education Department
Cultural Education Center
Albany, New York 12230
Tel: (518) 474-3817

NORTH CAROLINA
Executive Director
Board of Nursing
P.O. Box 2129
Raleigh, North Carolina 27602
Tel: (919) 828-0740

NORTH DAKOTA
Executive Director
Board of Nursing
418 East Rosser
Bismarck, North Dakota 58501
Tel: (701) 224-2974

OHIO
Executive Secretary
Board of Nursing Education and
  Nursing Registration
65 South Front Street
Suite 509
Columbus, Ohio 43215
Tel: (614) 466-3947

OKLAHOMA
Executive Director
Board of Nurse Registration and
  Nursing Education
2915 N. Classen Boulevard
Suite 524
Oklahoma City, Oklahoma 73106
Tel: (405) 525-2076

OREGON
Executive Director
Board of Nursing
1400 S.W. 5th Avenue, Room 904
Portland, Oregon 97201
Tel: (503) 229-5653

PENNSYLVANIA
Secretary
State Board of Nurse Examiners
Dept. of State, P.O. Box 2649
Harrisburg, Pennsylvania 17105
Tel: (717) 783-7146

RHODE ISLAND
Executive Secretary
Board of Nurse Registration
  and Nursing Education
Health Department Bldg.
75 Davis Street, Room 104
Providence, RI 02908-2488
Tel: (401) 277-2827

SOUTH CAROLINA
Executive Director
Board of Nursing for South Carolina
1777 St. Julian Pl., Suite 102
Columbia, South Carolina 29204
Tel: (803) 758-2611

SOUTH DAKOTA
Executive Secretary
Board of Nursing
304 S. Phillips Ave., Suite 205
Sioux Falls, South Dakota 57102
Tel: (605) 334-1243

TENNESSEE
Executive Director
State Board of Nursing
283 Plus Park Boulevard
Nashville, Tennessee 37219-5407
Tel: (615) 361-6705

TEXAS
Executive Secretary
Board of Nurse Examiners for
   the State of Texas
1300 Anderson Lane, Bldg. C
Suite 225
Austin, Texas 78752
Tel: (512) 835-4880

Executive Director
Board of Vocational Nurse
   Examiners
1300 Anderson Lane, Bldg. C
Suite 285
Austin, Texas 78752
Tel: (512) 835-2071

UTAH
Executive Secretary and
   Nurse Consultant
State Board of Nursing
Div. of Registration
Heber M. Wells Bldg., 4th Floor
160 East 300 South
P.O. Box 5802
Salt Lake City, Utah 84110
Tel: (801) 530-6638

VERMONT
Board of Nursing
Redstone Building
26 Terrace Street
Montpelier, Vermont 05602
Tel: (802) 828-3180

VIRGIN ISLANDS
Chairperson
Board of Nurse Licensure
Div. of Professional Licensing
P.O. Box 7309
Charlotte Amalie
St. Thomas, Virgin Islands 00801
Tel: (809) 774-9000, ext. 204

VIRGINIA
Executive Secretary
Board of Nursing
P.O. Box 27708
Richmond, Virginia 23261
Tel: (804) 786-0377

WASHINGTON
Executive Secretary
Board of Nursing
Div. of Professional Licensing
P.O. Box 9649
Olympia, Washington 98504
Tel: (206) 753-3726

Executive Secretary
State Board of Practical Nursing
P.O. Box 9649
Olympia, Washington 98504
Tel: (206) 753-3729

WEST VIRGINIA
Executive Secretary
Board of Examiners for
   Registered Nurses
922 Quarrier Street
Suite 309, Embleton Bldg.
Charleston, West Virginia 25301
Tel: (304) 348-3596

Executive Secretary
State Board of Examiners for
   Practical Nurses
922 Quarrier Street
Suite 506, Embleton Bldg.
Charleston, West Virginia 25301
Tel: (304) 348-3572

WISCONSIN
Director
Wisconsin Bureau of Nursing
Dept. of Regulation & Licensing
P.O. Box 8936
Madison, Wisconsin 53708
Tel: (608) 266-3735

WYOMING
Executive Director
Board of Nursing
2223 Warren Avenue
Suite 1 — 2nd Floor
Cheyenne, Wyoming 82002
Tel: (307) 777-7601

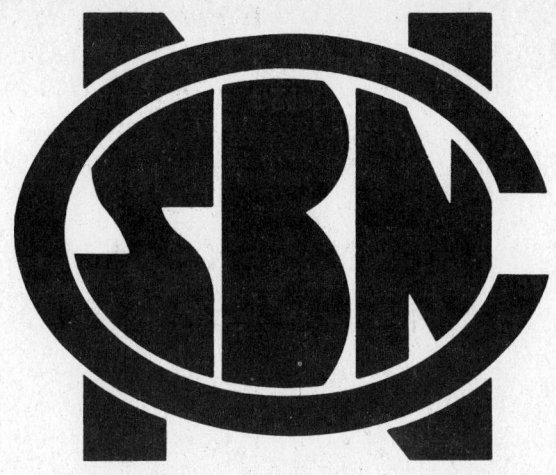

Test Plan for the National Council Licensure Examination for Practical Nurses

NATIONAL COUNCIL OF STATE BOARDS OF NURSING, INC.

October 1984

May be reproduced by state-approved schools of nursing for use in their educational programs. All other rights reserved.

© *1984* by the National Council of State Boards of Nursing, Inc.
625 N. Michigan   Suite 1544   Chicago, Illinois 60611

TEST PLAN FOR THE NATIONAL COUNCIL LICENSURE EXAMINATION FOR PRACTICAL NURSES

Introduction

Entry into the practice of practical nursing in the United States and its territories is regulated by the licensing authorities in the jurisdictions. Each jurisdiction requires a candidate for licensure to pass an examination that measures the competencies needed to perform safely and effectively as a newly licensed entry-level practical nurse.[1] Developed by the National Council of State Boards of Nursing, Inc., the National Council Licensure Examination for Practical Nurses is the examination used by those jurisdictions whose boards of nursing are National Council Members.

The initial step in developing the examination for practical nurse licensure was the preparation of a test plan to function as a guide for selecting content that represents the behaviors to be tested. The test plan reflects practical nursing practice as identified in the job analysis described in PRACTICAL NURSE ROLE DELINEATION AND VALIDATION STUDY FOR THE NATIONAL COUNCIL LICENSURE EXAMINATION FOR PRACTICAL NURSES (Ference 1983). The activities identified in the practical nurse job analysis were analyzed in relation to the complexity of managing data, the complexity of interrelating with people and the complexity of physically attending to objects or things required to perform the activity.[2] This process produced a competency model of entry-level practical nursing which includes practical nursing activities, content, and practice settings. The test plan, which was derived from the competency model, provides a concise summary of the content and scope of the examination and serves as a guide for the candidates preparing to write the examination and for those who develop it.

Structure of the Test Plan

The practical nurse test plan consists of three independently weighted scales: practical nursing activities, practice settings and age ranges of clients. These scales are related directly to the findings of the job analysis. There are eight categories of practical nursing activities which are weighted according to their criticality and frequency of performance and ranked according to complexity using the organizing framework of data, people and things. The categories and the range of percent of questions for each category included in the test plan are listed below in rank order with the first category representing the most complex activities.

Categories	Percent Range
I. Communicating and Participating in Plans of Care	3 to 7 %
II. Administering Special Therapies: Medications/Oxygen	13 to 17 %
III. Providing for Therapeutic Needs	18 to 22 %
IV. Providing for Basic Health Needs	8 to 12 %
V. Collecting and Recording Information	17 to 21 %
VI. Maintaining Safety	14 to 18 %
VII. Promoting Hygiene and Self Care	10 to 14 %
VIII. Maintaining a Healthy Environment	1 to 5 %

---

[1] *The job analysis identifies the entry level practical nurse as a newly licensed practical nurse who has been employed full time for less than seven months.*

[2] *United States Department of Labor, DICTIONARY OF OCCUPATIONAL TITLES. Washington, D.C.: Superintendent of Documents, 1965.*

Categories, Specific Activities, and Knowledge, Skills and Abilities

The eight categories of practical nursing activities are described below. The specific activities, which were identified by the job analysis, are listed in the respective categories in order of criticality and frequency. Also included are examples of knowledge, skills and abilities necessary to perform the activities.

I. COMMUNICATING AND PARTICIPATING IN PLANS OF CARE

The practical nurse participates as a member of the health care team in developing and evaluating plans of care, provides emotional support and guidance, implements health teaching as appropriate to the scope of practice, and communicates with clients and their significant others.

Activities

1.01 Obtaining Guidance for Difficult Communication
1.02 Instructing Clients on Health Promotion
1.03 Explaining the Reasons for a Procedure for Physical and Special Examinations
1.04 Care Planning with an RN
1.05 Explaining the Activities During a Procedure which is Part of a Physical or Special Examination
1.06 Evaluating Care Plans with an RN
1.07 Supporting the Family of the Dying Client
1.08 Providing Verbalization Time for the Dying Client
1.09 Obtaining Consent for Nursing Care
1.10 Instructing the Family About Transfers and Discharges
1.11 Assisting the RN in Teaching Tracheostomy Care

Knowledge, Skills and Abilities

In order to perform these activities, a candidate should possess knowledge, skills and abilities in areas which include but are not limited to the following examples: body structure and function; nursing process; basic human needs common to all individuals; principles of therapeutic communication; mental health concepts; basic teaching-learning principles; effect of the client's background, including age, occupation and family situation; and community agencies concerned with health maintenance.

II. ADMINISTERING SPECIAL THERAPIES: MEDICATIONS/OXYGEN

The practical nurse participates as a member of the health care team in administering prescribed medications and oxygen and monitoring intravenous therapy.

2.01 Administering Oral Medications
2.02 Withdrawing Medicine from Vials
2.03 Administering Intramuscular Injections
2.04 Administering Topical Medications
2.05 Withdrawing Medicine from Ampuls
2.06 Checking the Oxygen Flowmeter
2.07 Administering Subcutaneous Medications
2.08 Administering Suppository Medications
2.09 Turning on the Appropriate Liter Flow of Oxygen
2.10 Administering Eye Medications
2.11 Placing the Oxygen Apparatus

2.12 Selecting the Medication Route when **Two Are Prescribed**
2.13 Discontinuing Intravenous Needles
2.14 Recognizing Adverse Reactions to Intravenous Therapy
2.15 Administering Medication Soaks
2.16 Administering Ear Medications
2.17 Administering Nasal Medications
2.18 Administering Medications by Inhalation
2.19 Applying the Oxygen Delivery Device to the Client
2.20 Stopping an Intravenous Infusion
2.21 Administering Intradermal Injections for Immunizations
2.22 Regulating Intravenous Flow

Knowledge, Skills and Abilities

In order to perform these activities, a candidate should possess knowledge, skills and abilities in areas which include but are not limited to the following examples: therapeutic effects, side effects, and untoward effects of medications and oxygen used to treat commonly recurring health conditions; calculation of medication dosages; administration of medications and oxygen by appropriate methods and routes; body structure and function; signs of shock and oxygen deficiency; and medical and surgical asepsis.

III. PROVIDING FOR THERAPEUTIC NEEDS

The practical nurse participates as a member of the health care team in providing therapeutic and lifesaving procedures, prepares clients for surgery, cares for clients **postoperatively**, and assists clients in maintaining therapeutic regimens.

Activities
3.01 Giving Postoperative Care
3.02 Correcting Posture and **Balance During Ambulation**
3.03 Changing Sterile Dressings
3.04 Changing Surgical Dressings
3.05 Giving Preoperative Care
3.06 Applying Bandages
3.07 Catheterizing Female Urinary Tract
3.08 Checking Circulation During Cast Care
3.09 Applying Compresses
3.10 Removing Indwelling Catheters
3.11 Inserting Indwelling Catheters
3.12 Applying Soaks
3.13 Suctioning the Nasopharynx
3.14 Inducing **Deep-Breathing** Exercises
3.15 Inducing Coughing Exercises
3.16 Inserting Straight Urinary Catheters
3.17 Conducting Nasogastric Irrigations
3.18 Applying Binders
3.19 Conducting Intermittent Continuous Bladder Irrigations
3.20 Assisting with Walking with Walkers
3.21 Packing Deep Wounds
3.22 Applying Packs
3.23 Stimulating Urination
3.24 Catheterizing Male Urinary Tract

3.25 Irrigating Colostomies
3.26 Administering Cleansing Enemas
3.27 Removing Nasogastric Tubes
3.28 Preparing Skin for Aspetic Procedures
3.29 Administering Gastrostomy Feedings
3.30 Irrigating Wounds
3.31 Giving Ostomy Care
3.32 Assisting with Walking with Canes
3.33 Protecting Newly Applied Casts
3.34 Performing CPR
3.35 Maintaining Skeletal/Skin Traction
3.36 Covering Rough Edges of Dry Casts
3.37 Assisting with Walking with Crutches
3.38 Administering Gastric Gavage
3.39 Providing Tracheostomy Care
3.40 Providing Cystocatheter Care
3.41 Changing Tracheostomy Ties
3.42 Administering Oil-Retention Enemas
3.43 Conducting Postural Drainage
3.44 Irrigating the Vagina
3.45 Assisting with Walking with Braces
3.46 Irrigating the Throat and Mouth
3.47 Administering Medicated Retention Enemas
3.48 Irrigating Eyes
3.49 Maintaining Patency of Tubes
3.50 Conducting Endotracheal Suctioning

Knowledge, Skills and Abilities

In order to perform these activities, a candidate should possess knowledge, skills and abilities in areas which include but are not limited to the following examples: therapeutic and untoward effects of heat and cold; body structure and function; signs and symptoms of shock, hemorrhage and infection; medical and surgical asepsis; and factors that promote wound healing.

IV. PROVIDING FOR BASIC HEALTH NEEDS

The practical nurse participates as a member of the health care team in providing therapies, hygiene and nutritional needs, and supporting and adjusting the client's body.

Activities
4.01 Positioning and Turning
4.02 Reducing Pressure Areas
4.03 Supporting Body Parts
4.04 Assisting Clients In and Out of Bed
4.05 Conducting Range of Motion Exercises
4.06 Massaging Pressure Areas
4.07 Administering Perineal Care
4.08 Applying Heating Pads
4.09 Applying Ice Applications
4.10 Evaluating Suitability of Food
4.11 Assisting with Showers
4.12 Applying Heating Lamps

4.13 Making Occupied Beds
4.14 Giving Partial Baths
4.15 Giving Tub Baths
4.16 Giving Complete Baths
4.17 Inserting Rectal Tubes
4.18 Giving Alcohol or Tepid Baths for Systemic Temperature Modification
4.19 Giving Tepid Baths for Local Temperature Modification
4.20 Giving Sitz Baths
4.21 Helping Clients Select Food
4.22 Interpreting the Nutritional Value of Foods

Knowledge, Skills and Abilities

In order to perform these activities, a candidate should possess knowledge, skills and abilities in areas which include but are not limited to the following examples: heat-regulating mechanism; principles of proper body mechanics; maintenance of healthy skin and avoidance of factors contributing to skin breakdown; principles of correct body alignment; appropriate comfort measures; principles of normal nutrition; and dietary modifications for commonly recurring health conditions.

V. COLLECTING AND RECORDING INFORMATION

The practical nurse measures and records client's baseline data; assists in special examinations and procedures; and collects specimens.

Activities
5.01 Recording Measurements Such as TPR
5.02 Measuring Respirations
5.03 Measuring Radial Rates
5.04 Measuring and Recording Output
5.05 Measuring and Recording Intake
5.06 Measuring Apical Rates
5.07 Measuring Temperatures
5.08 Recording Measurements
5.09 Writing Nurses Notes
5.10 Measuring Apical/Radial Rates
5.11 Measuring Pedal Pulses
5.12 Observing Client's Neurological Functioning,
    including level of consciousness and pupillary reactions
5.13 Recording Miscellaneous Specimens
5.14 Obtaining Specimens for Urine Culture
5.15 Measuring Femoral Pulses
5.16 Measuring Weight
5.17 Measuring Fetal Heart Rates
5.18 Measuring Shock Symptoms
5.19 Measuring Height
5.20 Obtaining Specimens for Wound Culture
5.21 Obtaining Specimens for Throat Culture
5.22 Measuring Sight
5.23 Obtaining Specimens for Skin Culture
5.24 Auscultating Breath Sounds
5.25 Obtaining Specimens for Nose Culture
5.26 Assisting Physicians with Procedures

5.27 Obtaining Specimens for Vaginal Cultures
5.28 Recording that a Procedure is Done
5.29 Measuring Hearing
5.30 Assisting Physicians with Neurological Examinations
5.31 Assessing Cardiac Status

Knowledge, Skills and Abilities

In order to perform these activities, a candidate should possess knowledge, skills and abilities in areas which include but are not limited to the following examples: signs and symptoms of major health problems; factors predisposing to illness; purposes of special examinations; client's response to illness; body structure and function; differentiation between normal and abnormal responses; legal aspects of patient's record; and principles of charting.

VI. MAINTAINING SAFETY

The practical nurse maintains sterile and aseptic technique and provides for the client's safety and rights.

Activities
6.01 Handwashing
6.02 Positioning Side Rails/Bed Height
6.03 Placing Signal Cords
6.04 Maintaining Safety from Fire
6.05 Insuring that Client's Rights are Honored
6.06 Opening Sterile Gloves
6.07 Applying Restraints
6.08 Applying Sterile Gloves
6.09 Transcribing Prescriptions/Orders
6.10 Observing Client's Bill of Rights
6.11 Self-gloving
6.12 Pouring Sterile Solutions
6.13 Maintaining Isolation
6.14 Grasping a Falling Client
6.15 Operating Special Beds
6.16 Adding Water to Oxygen Humidifiers
6.17 Self-gowning
6.18 Assessing Food Allergies
6.19 Positioning Clients on Side During Seizure
6.20 Moving Nearby Objects During Seizure
6.21 Calling for Help During Seizure
6.22 Transferring Sterile Forceps
6.23 Enforcing Hospital Regulations
6.24 Informing Clients of Evacuation Procedures
6.25 Monitoring Seizure Patterns
6.26 Surgical Scrubbing

Knowledge, Skills and Abilities

In order to perform these activities, a candidate should possess knowledge, skills and abilities in areas which include but are not limited to the following examples: medical and surgical asepsis; spread of infectious diseases; isolation techniques, theories of combustion and elimination of fire hazards; client's bill of rights; hazards of immobility; seizure patterns and seizure precautions; body mechanics; and fire and disaster plans.

VII. PROMOTING HYGIENE AND SELF-CARE

The practical nurse assists the client in activities of daily living; performs basic hygienic measures for the client when necessary; and orients the client to the environment.

Activities
7.01 Using Transportation Equipment
7.02 Applying Lotion to Skin
7.03 Assisting Clients to Use Bedpans
7.04 Assisting Clients with Elimination/Bathroom
7.05 Assisting Clients to Use Urinals
7.06 Transferring Clients Out of Bed
7.07 Administering Mouth Care
7.08 Assisting Clients to Use Bedside Commode
7.09 Giving Between-Meal Feedings
7.10 Removing Irritants from the Environment
7.11 Transferring Clients Within an Agency
7.12 Feeding Adult Clients
7.13 Changing Clothing
7.14 Orienting to Surroundings
7.15 Giving Backrubs
7.16 Positioning Clients for Meals
7.17 Explaining Hospital Regulations
7.18 Cleansing Clients Between Baths
7.19 Combing Client's Hair
7.20 Informing About the Hospital and Personnel
7.21 Shaving Clients
7.22 Transferring or Discharging Clients Outside of the Agency
7.23 Shampooing Hair
7.24 Providing Postmortem Care

Knowledge, Skills and Abilities

In order to perform these activities, a candidate should possess knowledge, skills and abilities in areas which include but are not limited to the following examples: comfort and hygiene measures; activities of daily living; normal nutrition; elimination patterns; principles of body mechanics; and principles of communication and interpersonal relations.

VIII. MAINTAINING A HEALTHY ENVIRONMENT

The practical nurse prepares the client's environment by maintaining and cleaning equipment and supplies; and provides for the safe-keeping of the client's possessions.

Activities
8.01 Storing Stock Drugs
8.02 Checking Emergency Equipment
8.03 Checking Emergency Supplies
8.04 Making Unoccupied Beds
8.05 Cleaning Equipment and Utensils
8.06 Making Anesthetic/Surgical Beds

8.07 Serving or Collecting Food Trays
8.08 Sterilizing Equipment and Supplies
8.09 Cleaning the Clinical Unit Service Areas
8.10 Inventorying Client's Possessions
8.11 Cleaning Rooms
8.12 Storing Client's Possessions in a Safe Place
8.13 Checking Stock Equipment Function
8.14 Cleaning Furniture
8.15 Conducting Terminal Disinfection

Knowledge, Skills and Abilities

In order to perform these activities, a candidate should possess knowledge, skills and abilities in areas which include but are not limited to the following examples: medical and surgical asepsis; principles of proper waste disposal; effects of sensory overload; client's bill of rights; environmental controls; purpose of emergency supplies; and functioning of emergency equipment.

Practice Settings and Age Ranges

The percent of questions that relate to specific practice settings and to the age ranges of clients follow the findings as described in the job analysis. These weightings are used in developing the clinical situations for the examination. The percent of questions representing the various types of practice settings and the age ranges of clients are presented below.

Practice Settings	Percent Range
Acute Care Settings	65 to 75 %
Extended Care Settings	15 to 25 %
Ambulatory Care Settings	5 to 15 %

Age Ranges of Clients	Percent Range
Birth to 19 Years	5 to 15 %
20 to 65 Years	55 to 65 %
66 Years and Older	25 to 35 %

Categories of Human Functioning

In order to provide a structure for the content to be tested in the examination, the theoretical model of human functioning is used. The human functioning model explains the major alterations that occur during illness. Nursing activities, organized within the framework of the nursing process, are performed in situations that include one of the categories of human functioning. The categories of human functioning are described below. Although these categories are used to organize the content, no specific weight for each category is assigned.

1. **Protective Functions**

    The client's capacity or ability to maintain defenses and prevent physical and chemical trauma, injury, infection, and threats to health status.

    Examples: Nursing care situations and nursing measures which include but are not limited to the following content areas: communicable diseases (including sexually transmitted diseases), immunizations, physical trauma and abuse, asepsis, safety hazards, poisoning, skin disorders, preoperative care, and postoperative complications.

2. **Sensory-Perceptual Functions**

   The client's capacity or ability to be aware of stimuli, understand stimuli and respond to stimuli.

   Examples: Nursing care situations and nursing measures which include but are not limited to the following content areas: auditory, visual and verbal impairments, sensory deprivation, aphasia, brain tumors, laryngectomy, organic brain syndrome, body image, reality orientation, cerebral vascular accident, and seizure disorders.

3. **Comfort, Rest, Activity and Mobility**

   The client's capacity or ability to maintain mobility, a desirable level of activity, and adequate sleep, rest and comfort.

   Examples: Nursing care situations and nursing measures which include but are not limited to the following content areas: joint impairment, body alignment, pain, sleep disturbances, activities of daily living, neuromuscular impairment, musculoskeletal impairment, and endocrine disorders that affect activity.

4. **Nutrition**

   The client's capacity or ability to maintain the intake and processing of essential nutrients.

   Examples: Nursing care situations and nursing measures which include but are not limited to the following content areas: normal nutrition, diet in pregnancy and lactation, obesity, and conditions such as diabetes, gastric disorders, and metabolic disorders that primarily affect the nutritional status.

5. **Growth and Development**

   The client's capacity or ability to maintain maturational processess occuring throughout the life span.

   Examples: Nursing care situations and nursing measures which include but are not limited to the following content areas: childbearing, child rearing, normal physical growth and development throughout the life cycle, conditions that interfere with the maturation process or create crises, and changes in aging, sterility, and conditions of the reproductive system.

6. **Fluid-Gas Transport**

   The client's capacity or ability to maintain fluid-gas transport.

   Examples: Nursing care situations and nursing measures which include but are not limited to the following content areas: cardio-pulmonary diseases, cardio-pulmonary resuscitation, anemias, hemorrhagic disorders, leukemias, infectious pulmonary diseases, dehydration, and edema.

7. **Psycho-Socio-Cultural Functions**

   The client's capacity or ability to function in intrapersonal, interpersonal, intergroup and socio-cultural relationships.

   Examples: Nursing care situations and nursing measures which include but are not limited to the following content areas: grieving, death and dying, substance abuse, self-concept, general community resources, spiritual needs, life crises, gross signs of emotional and mental health, gross signs of development, and basic principles of interpersonal communication.

8. **Elimination**

The client's capacity or ability to maintain functions related to relieving the body of waste products.

Examples: Nursing care situations and nursing measures which include but are not limited to the following content areas: conditions of the gastro-intestinal system such as vomiting, diarrhea, constipation, ulcers, neoplasms, colostomy, ileostomy, and hernia. Conditions of the urinary system such as kidney stones, neoplasms, renal failure, and prostatic hypertrophy.

BIBLIOGRAPHY

Ference, Helen M. PRACTICAL NURSE ROLE DELINEATION AND VALIDATION STUDY FOR THE NATIONAL COUNCIL LICENSURE EXAMINATION FOR PRACTICAL NURSES. Monterey, CA: CTB/McGraw-Hill, 1983.

United States Department of Labor. DICTIONARY OF OCCUPATIONAL TITLES. Washington, D.C.: Superintendent of Documents, 1965.